A Hot Mess

Tips, Tricks and Truths About
Menopause and Perimenopause

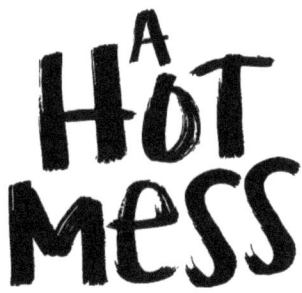

Tips, Tricks and Truths About
Menopause and Perimenopause

BARBARA ANN HANNAH, MD, MS, FACOG

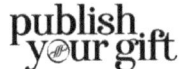

A HOT MESS
Copyright © 2021 Barbara Ann Hannah
All rights reserved.

Published by Publish Your Gift®
An imprint of Purposely Created Publishing Group, LLC

No part of this book may be reproduced, distributed or transmitted in any form by any means, graphic, electronic, or mechanical, including photocopy, recording, taping, or by any information storage or retrieval system, without permission in writing from the publisher, except in the case of reprints in the context of reviews, quotes, or references.

Printed in the United States of America

ISBN: 978-1-64484-387-1 (print)
ISBN: 978-1-64484-388-8 (ebook)

Special discounts are available on bulk quantity purchases by book clubs, associations and special interest groups. For details email: sales@publishyourgift.com or call (888) 949-6228.
For information log on to www.PublishYourGift.com

Once I began to look to myself, I began to realize that the wizard of Oz is inside of me.

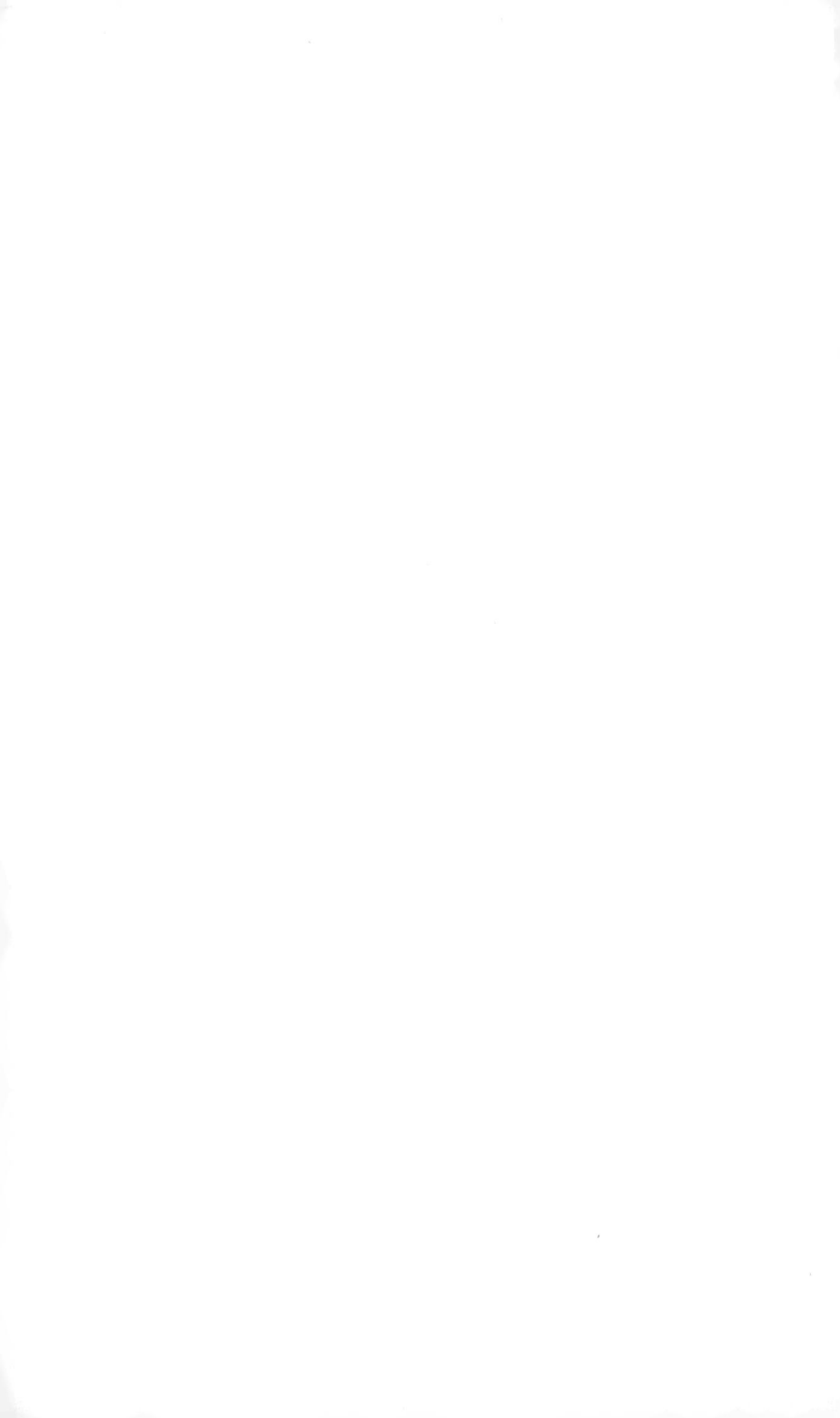

DEDICATION

༄

Although they are no longer here in the physical sense, my parents, John and Elizabeth Hannah, continue to inspire me from the heavenly realm. While on earth, they believed in me before I knew who I was. They knew the potential I had to become whatever GOD designed me to be and they nurtured that potential. They set the course in action and gave me the necessary tools to move forward. To them, I dedicate this book.

To my husband, my best friend, my soul mate, my life partner and the wind beneath my wings, James Henry Kerns, III. You were there when I struggled to complete this manuscript. You buoyed me with your words when I needed, and you gave me silence when I didn't. Your LOVE renders me unstoppable because, with it, I have no limitations. You challenge me to the next level. Your strength leads to my glory. This manuscript is possible because you are in my life.

To my forefathers and foremothers, the progenitors of all humankind, the origin of all human civilization, I salute you. We never met, but your blood courses through my veins. You could not imagine beyond the sear of the branding iron. You could not dream beyond the lash of the whip. The excruciating toil of your day is unimaginable. I see your pain as well as your resilience. I am because you were. I dedicate this book to you, your impossible dreams and your suppressed desires that were not allowed to come to pass. I am here to say thank you, and wherever you rest in the heavens, know that you will always be remembered.

TABLE OF CONTENTS

Foreword by Dr. Drai xi

Introduction 1

Chapter 1: Menopausal Basics 5

Chapter 2: The Reproductive System on Menopause 11

Chapter 3: The Endocrine and Urinary Systems on Menopause 19

Chapter 4: The Nervous and Cardiovascular Systems on Menopause 31

Chapter 5: The Integumentary and Digestive Systems on Menopause 37

Chapter 6: The Respiratory and Musculoskeletal Systems on Menopause 43

Chapter 7: The Immune System on Menopause 49

Chapter 8: Treatment of Menopausal Symptoms, Part I 53

Chapter 9: Treatment of Menopausal Symptoms, Part II 69

Chapter 10: Nutrition, Exercise, and Lifestyle Changes in Menopause 79

Chapter 11: The Doctor's Visit 87
Chapter 12: Menopause and Medication 95
Chapter 13: The Best of Menopause 105
The Menopausal Quiz 109
My Menopausal Guide 117
Afterword 123
Acknowledgments 125
References 127
About the Author 129

FOREWORD

Dear Ladies,

Are you a woman who is having hot flashes, mood swings, or trouble sleeping? Are you a woman who is having painful sex and/or who doesn't want to have sex at all? Are you a woman who has gained weight and can't seem to lose it no matter what? If you answered YES to ANY of these questions, this book is just for you. In this book, Dr. Barbara teaches you all the things you need to know in order to manage these symptoms during the most important time of a woman's life: menopause.

Ladies, close your eyes and imagine what the world would be like if you woke up without wet sheets, were always in a happy mood, slept well throughout the night, wanted to have pleasurable sex, and lost weight when eating a balanced diet and routinely exercising. Dr. Barbara is going to teach you how. Keep reading.

As an obstetrician and gynecologist, Dr. Barbara has had the privilege of taking care of female patients with a myriad of obstetrical and gynecological issues. Her patients range in age from nine to ninety-nine and they come with a host of all types of concerns. Dr. Barbara is known in the medical field for her expertise in managing menopause.

Once you finish reading, you will understand how your body changes and what steps can help alleviate the symptoms of menopause.

Let me introduce myself. I'm Dr. Drai, board-certified OBGYN, eight-time bestselling author, international speaker, award-winning business coach, founder of the first FDA-approved condom and personal lubricant line created by a physician in the USA, and dean of an online B-school for medical professionals. I help doctors walk in their purpose, serve humanity in a big way, and have the time freedom that they deserve. I was so honored when Dr. Barbara asked me to write her foreword.

I met Dr. Barbara in April 2020 during my conference Momentum in Medicine. This is a conference for doctors to learn how to make a bigger impact on the world through medicine. When engaging with Dr. Barbara she stated she wanted to be the change agent globally for women suffering with symptoms of menopause. WOW! She joined our online B-school to help her start building and implementing her global mission. To date, Dr. Barbara Hannah has transformed more than 10,000 women's lives. And there's so many more lives waiting—yours included!

In this book, Dr. Barbara gives you a system that you can follow to take your life back. Ladies, don't let menopause manage your life. You have to manage it. Read this book more than once. Buy a copy for your girlfriends who also may need help slaying the symptoms of menopause. And to Dr. Barbara: Thank you for sharing your GIFT with the world. I'm so proud of you.

XOXO,
Dr. Drai, Dean of Medical Moguls Academy

INTRODUCTION

I am an artist who became a doctor. Since my elementary school days, I have loved to read and write the written word. I remember sitting in high school journalism class and envisioning myself as a writer for a large newspaper. Upon high school graduation, I began to grapple with my love of writing and my fascination for the human body. I loved the science classes and before I knew it, medicine as a career had beaten out writing.

I followed my dream of becoming a physician and it has been both grueling and gratifying. Fast forward to 2020, I was introduced to the Medical Moguls Academy where Dr. Draion Burch and his colleagues teach physicians to be the best they can be beyond the brick and mortar of the medical office. Voilá! The writing juices began to flow again, and I realized that there is a lot I can do beyond the basic medical practice and the brick and mortar of the medical office. I have an obligation to give back to the world what GOD has given me. To whom much is given, much is required.

As a practicing obstetrician and gynecologist, I see all types of patients from the prepubescent girl to the seasoned centenarian. However, it is the middle-aged woman that I have found the most joy in providing care for. Women come to me full of misconceptions they have been taught regarding menopause, inappropriate treatments they have endured and confused thoughts about the next phase they are entering. I felt that these women needed an advocate and I decided to be that person.

When we are young, we have no concept of what it means to age. During our younger years, we watch the aging people in our lives as they grow older and meet the challenges associated with aging. However, it is not until we board that train ourselves that the aging process takes on a new meaning for us. There are profound changes that occur as we age. Some we may embrace, while there may be others that we dislike and feel that we simply must endure. We can be certain that if we live long enough, these changes will happen. My mother used to say that we have only two choices when it comes to aging: "we are either old or cold." Since most of us would rather be old than cold, we may as well make the best of our aging years.

Women are beginning to realize that menopause needs to be discussed. A previously taboo subject is finally being seen as what it has always been—a normal, biological life phase. However, despite this there are still so few resources for women experiencing this transition. Recently, while watching a morning show, I saw an advertisement for a new menopausal product. The inventor of the product revealed how she had unlimited options in choosing a website domain name because so few sites relating to menopause and middle-aged women existed. The paucity of information and products available is astonishing. It is time to provide middle-aged women with the tools to make this transition a vibrant and confident one—and that is the intent of this book. Throughout the book, I have included the most common comments and concerns from my patients that pertain to different issues. You may find these relatable as you go through your menopausal journey.

This book is dedicated to the woman who wants to make the most of her aging years and who wants to be that dynamic, confident, and self-assured woman she was intended to be. This book is for that woman who needs some pointers on how to understand and accept the process that is occurring in her body. This book is for the woman who wants to make the most of the changes in her life as she ages. This book is for the woman who has entered what has the potential to be the most satisfying and productive years of her life. She is confident, dynamic, bold, and happy. This book is an oasis for her.

CHAPTER I

MENOPAUSAL BASICS

"I had premature menopause at age thirty-two and I had not had babies. I felt so cheated."

The change of life. The word change in and of itself is enough to send dread into the hearts of many women and their families. If we have not yet entered "the change," we have family members, coworkers, or friends who are going through or have gone through it. We hear stories about their "private summers" where the hot flashes are overwhelming and they want to strip themselves of the excess clothing in an attempt to cool down. Depending upon the comfort level of the woman, we may hear about the vaginal dryness and the decreased libido that she is wrestling with.

There is not a child of a menopausal woman who is foreign to the mood swings that plague their loved one. I can remember my mother in one moment being a wonderful and kind soul and in the next moment screaming her head off with no apparent provocation. My father and I would just look at one another and shake our heads. He later told me at the tender age of ten that all women go through the change. It meant virtually nothing to me at that time, until one day . . .

Menopause in the United States has been associated with dread and negativity. Just the word *menopause* conjures up a picture of a shriveled, brittle old woman yelling and screaming at the top of her lungs with no desire to have sexual relations. We don't want to be in her presence most days because we don't know the triggers that will set her off. We promise ourselves that when that time comes for us we will be different and we will not let this thing called menopause do to us what it is doing to that "poor soul over there."

The dread and negativity associated with menopause are NOT universal. I have traveled extensively and have noticed that in cultures where aging is celebrated, menopause is viewed through a different lens. These societies view it as a time of renewal and reinvigoration. The women have completed their childbearing and see menopause as the next stage in life to be enjoyed and celebrated. They see it as a time to embrace themselves and to rediscover who they are. They seek to have a deeper level of intimacy with their mates. As women in these societies age, they are viewed as wise counsel and find themselves to be the confidante and adviser of younger women. They revere themselves and are revered.

So why is their belief system different than that of Americans? I believe that it begins with our perception of the aging process. In the US, we are excited about and celebrate youth. In fact, I would say that our culture is obsessed with it. The media is flooded with pictures of young people, and there are all types of products on the market to help us maintain our youth and vitality. As we go through life, we unknowingly buy into this concept and believe that trying to hold onto our youth is what we must do. It is only within the past few years that we are beginning to celebrate the aging process in this country. Phrases such as "fifty is the new forty" can be seen in the media now. We see people working at their careers longer well into the seventh and eighth decade of life. It is about time that the United States got on board with other cultures and began to celebrate the aging process. Granted, some of the changes associated with the aging process are unpleasant, however, do we have a choice? We can either accept the changes and make the most of them, or we can just shrivel up and refuse to live the rest of our lives as the dynamic souls that we are.

As women age, the number of eggs in our ovaries begins to decrease and hormone production declines. The decline in ovarian function can happen as early as age thirty-five; however, the average age at, which ovarian function begins to decline is forty-five. This time period is known as perimenopause or around menopause. During perimenopause, the decline in ovarian function can bring about a multitude of symptoms including mood swings, depression, water weight gain, bloating, irregular menstrual cycles, and insomnia. Ovulation, the release of an egg from the ovaries, happens less frequently, but because it can still happen, pregnancy in the perimenopausal woman is still possible. The oldest patient I delivered was forty-nine years old and the patient did well and the baby came out fat and fine!

The time period of perimenopause can last for up to ten years, often from age forty-five to fifty-five. The average age of menopause in the United States is 52.4 years. Menopause, defined as the complete cessation of menses for a full year, can bring about a host of symptoms. There is as much variation in menopausal symptoms as there are women on earth. Some women will breeze through the change while other women will have every symptom known to womankind. Also, the length of time that a patient will have symptoms is also as varied as the patient herself. I have seen some patients grapple with symptoms well into their seventies and eighties while others are essentially symptom free. Every system of the body is affected by menopause, so the symptoms associated with this time of life can be numerous.

Although menopause has been a part of life since the beginning of time, our mothers and grandmothers rarely discussed it. However, as their children and grandchildren, we knew that something was different about them. They were short tempered, more than usual. We could catch them crying for no apparent reason. They never seemed to be able to get comfortable because their internal thermostat was always in a constant flux. Since menopause was rarely discussed, few treatment options were known. Women seemed to ignore this period of life and wanted to get through it as painlessly as possible.

Well things have changed, and now menopause is front and center. Through this book, I hope to encourage women to not only understand the bodily changes but to embrace them with solutions and options that allow this transition to be one of vibrancy, confidence, and renewal.

"You must do the thing you think you cannot do."

—ELEANOR ROOSEVELT

CHAPTER 2

THE REPRODUCTIVE SYSTEM ON MENOPAUSE

"I just don't know when my period is coming. I am so tired of taking a change of clothing with me. When I think I am done, well let's just say I carry extra underwear in my purse."

If the body is fascinating, the female reproductive system is a miraculous wonder. The internal anatomy of the reproductive system including its two ovaries, one uterus, two fallopian tubes, and one vagina has been a fascination of mankind for eons. The brain is the great orchestrator of the reproductive system. While the ovaries produce eggs and hormones, the fallopian tubes serve as the location of fertilization of the egg and the conduit to carry the fertilized egg to the uterus where it will be housed for approximately ten months. During these ten months, the fetus develops and is finally expelled through the vagina or birth canal into the waiting arms of the world. The brain acts as a conductor or the influencer of the process by navigating and orchestrating this miracle.

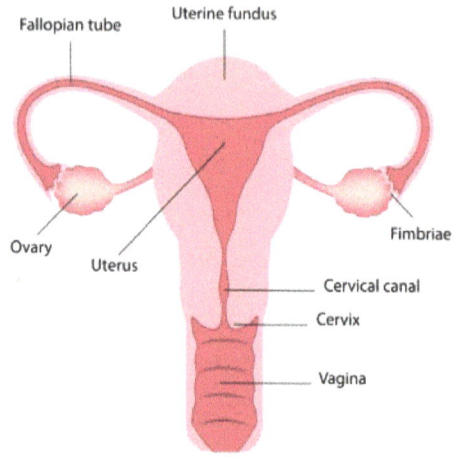

Female reproductive system

Before birth, the ovaries contain millions of eggs with the potential to become human beings. While we are developing in the uterus of our mothers, our bodies are developing their own eggs. This means that when females are born, they have all the follicles they will have for their lifetime. This number is estimated to be approximately two million, and by the time females reach puberty, those millions of eggs that were present during our in-utero experience have dwindled down to approximately 400,000. With each monthly menstrual cycle, we lose eggs in the process. This release of an egg from the ovary, termed ovulation, generally occurs once per month. When there are only about 1,000 eggs remaining in the ovaries, the process of ovulation rarely occurs and a woman can be said to be preparing for menopause.

While the production of eggs to make humans is fascinating enough, the ovaries also function to make female hormones. They are not the only organs that make female hormones, but they are by far where the majority of female hormones are made. Hormones are powerful chemical signals in the bloodstream that allow one organ to speak to another organ or organs. I find this part of medical science to be truly fascinating in that our organs, which may not be located in proximity to one another, have the ability to speak to each other via the endocrine system.

Multiple hormones or signals are produced in the female body and are derived from cholesterol. Despite the fact that we have been told that cholesterol can be bad, it is quite necessary because, without it, our bodies would not be able to make some of its hormones.

During the reproductive years, our bodies are in constant preparation to bring forth life. At puberty, BPAM happens. BPAM is the acronym for breast development, pubic hair development, axillary hair development, and menses. These events normally happen in that order. On average, the menstrual cycle begins at 12.8 years and can last for upwards of 40 years. During these years the ovaries release several eggs monthly with one of those eggs having the potential to become a human being while the other eggs are released in support of that one egg. Over the years, the supply of approximately 400,000 eggs that were present at puberty declines along with a subsequent decline in hormonal levels. With this decline in hormone production, the constellation of signs and symptoms associated with menopause begins. Can we say that every organ in the body is affected by the menopausal transition? YES, we can say that perimenopause and menopause affect every part of the body.

With the decline in ovarian reserve as well as hormonal decline, the once every twenty-eight-day bleeding becomes more and more irregular. The bleeding interval typically lengthens, and menses are more infrequent. Although the interval lengthening is a common bleeding pattern, other irregularities that occur include bleeding in between menses along with menses lasting longer than normal. The menstrual intervals continue to lengthen until the menses eventually stop. After twelve months of no menstrual flow, a woman is said to be in menopause.

One of the most common complaints of my transitioning women is the complaint of vaginal dryness. During our youthful years, estrogen is responsible for the plump, lubricated, and thick vaginal tissue. Additionally, the normal vagina is the home of multiple species of bacteria that help to protect the vagina from the "bad invaders" or bacteria that mean the vagina no good. The lining of the vagina, termed the vaginal mucosa or epithelium, is able to respond to sexual signals by secreting more fluids in preparation for sexual activity. Additionally, the youthful vagina has folds called rugae that help to increase friction during sexual intercourse. The thicker vaginal epithelium helps to make the younger vagina more resistant to invasion by both bacteria and viruses. Vaginas vary in length with the average length being between three and seven inches. With sexual arousal, the vagina lengthens. The vagina is acidic with a pH between 3.8 and 4.5, which also contributes to the vagina being a self-cleansing organ. What is significant about this? With this pH range, the beneficial bacteria are predominant and help to keep the negative bacteria in check. Estrogen also helps to maintain the external genitalia, the vulva, keeping it supple and strong.

In the perimenopausal/menopausal state, the vaginal epithelium undergoes changes due to the diminished levels of estrogen. This results in the vaginal epithelium becoming drier, thinner, and less flexible. More women experience these vaginal symptoms than do not. This process, known as vaginal atrophy, can begin as early as age forty. Another phenomenon in women who don't or rarely have sexual intercourse is the shortening and narrowing of the vaginal canal. Additionally, the menopausal vagina—because of its now thinner epithelium—is more prone to bacterial growth due to microscopic tears. There is an increase in vaginal itching and burning during these years. Bleeding during intercourse is common. The multiple changes that occur in the vagina are collectively termed atrophic vaginitis. Vaginal atrophy is one of the most common causes of vaginal discharge in the postmenopausal patient. The now thinner and less elastic vaginal epithelium secretes a thin, watery discharge. Patients may assume that there is some type of infectious process going on and seek medical advice.

The decline in estrogen leads to a decrease in pubic hair resulting in a more smooth and hairless vulva. The hair becomes grayer just like the hair on the head. The tissue can become itchy as well and more susceptible to allergic reactions. Other changes that can occur in the external genitalia include color changes where the skin can either darken significantly or lighten.

Still other changes occur in the external genitalia anatomy. There is a decrease in the production of fluid from the surrounding vestibular glands during sexual arousal, which contributes to more painful and drier intercourse. The clitoris, the exquisitely sensitive pea-sized gland located at the area where the labia minora meet, has thousands of nerve endings that contribute to it being a primary erogenous zone. During sexual arousal, it swells to almost double its size. As women transition into the change, the clitoris becomes smaller and the organ that used to bring so much pleasure can now bring so much pain.

During our younger years, the mons pubis (the area that sports the pubic hair) is a soft and fatty mound of tissue. With the aging process, the pubic hair begins to recede as does the fat that is part of the mons pubis. With this decrease in the fat, the area becomes to take on an elongated appearance and is given the term "the hanging vagina." In reality, this area is not actually hanging, but the loss of subcutaneous fat gives it the appearance that it is.

The female breasts are part of both the reproductive system as well as the integumentary system. The breasts are constantly undergoing changes from the in-utero breasts to the menopausal breasts. While in the uterus, a milk line develops in the chest area of the female fetus and represents where the breasts will be. At birth, the female infant has developed nipples and the milk duct system has formed. During the teen years, visible signs of breast development occur. The breasts begin to enlarge as the increase in fat cells occurs and the duct system develops. Glands and lobules begin to develop. During pregnancy and as milk production begins, the breasts continue to undergo changes. The changes in the pregnant breast happen early in the pregnancy due to the hormone progesterone. The areola darkens and the breasts become swollen. More lobules are forming in the breasts during this time, which often leads to breast soreness and tenderness.

Changes occur in the menopausal breast as well. With the decline of estrogen and progesterone, supportive connective tissue of the breasts becomes less pliable and the breasts begin to sag. The breasts lose shape and begin to droop. Another change that occurs in the menopausal breast is breast tenderness. My menopausal patients are concerned about this breast pain, termed *mastalgia*, and wonder about the risk of breast cancer. Of note, breast pain is rarely associated with breast cancer.

"If I didn't define myself for myself, I would be crunched into other people's fantasies for me and eaten alive."

—AUDRE LORDE

CHAPTER 3

THE ENDOCRINE AND URINARY SYSTEMS ON MENOPAUSE

"I hate the lack of control I have as I go through this change. The night sweats have me getting up in the middle of the night and my pajamas are soaked."

THE ENDOCRINE SYSTEM

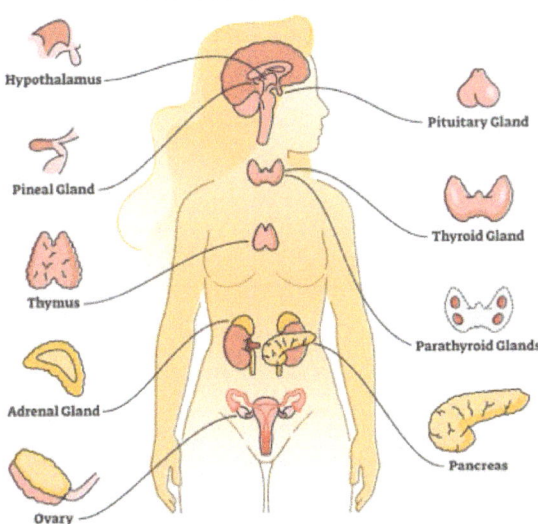

The endocrine system orchestrates multiple functions including growth and development, mood stabilization, metabolism, sexual function, and reproduction. It does so by utilizing tiny molecules called hormones, or chemical messengers, that travel through the bloodstream being released by one organ and traveling to another organ to influence its function. Upon being released by one organ, the hormone will attach to another organ's surface, allowing organs to speak to one another. A well-functioning endocrine system is like a symphony that helps to control functions such as heart rate, blood pressure, sleep cycles, appetite, and body temperature. Hormonal levels and function are greatly affected during perimenopause and menopause.

Insomnia

At least half of my menopausal patients complain of the inability to fall asleep or stay asleep. Insomnia affects us tremendously with long-standing consequences. Chronic sleep deprivation can cause serious conditions such as hypertension, heart attacks, depression, and a decrease in the efficacy of the immune system. Insomnia also causes a decreased ability to concentrate, poor memory, drowsiness, and an increase in mood swings. Premature wrinkles and under-eye dark circles are worsened with sleep deprivation.

There are various reasons for menopausal insomnia. One of the major reasons is the decrease in the production of the hormone melatonin. Melatonin, which is involved in the sleep-wake cycle and secreted by the pineal gland, decreases with age. With less melatonin production, insomnia is more common. Additionally, hot flashes and night sweats caused by the decreases in estrogen and progesterone interrupt sleep. These sleep disturbances further increase mood swings and irritability, which in turn worsen the insomnia. It becomes a vicious cycle. Sleep disturbances also occur as a result of urinary frequency associated with menopause.

Once thought to be a disease of men, sleep apnea has been found to affect women too, especially during the perimenopause/menopause transition. While there are a vast number of hormones in the human body, the sex steroid hormones play a very significant role in the female. I call these hormones "the big three" or the "female trifecta." These hormones are derived from cholesterol making an appropriate and adequate amount of cholesterol necessary for hormone production.

The trifecta of female hormones include testosterone, estrogen, and progesterone. Testosterone is part of a group of hormones called androgens. It may come as a surprise that women too have testosterone. Although women have far less testosterone than men, the smaller quantities found in women are important in maintaining the musculoskeletal system and red blood cell production. Testosterone also helps control sexual desire and provides a feeling of overall well-being.

The second trifecta hormone is estrogen. Estrogen is responsible for the pubertal growth spurt and development of the female sexual characteristics. During the reproductive years, estrogen is produced primarily by the ovaries, but once menopause occurs, estrogen comes primarily from muscle, skin, and fat cells.

Progesterone is the third part of the trifecta. Secreted by the ovaries, adrenal glands, and the pregnant placenta, this hormone is responsible for maintaining pregnancy and fertility. It also functions to facilitate urination, provides a calming effect, and is involved with cholesterol metabolism and sexual desire.

Sexual Health

This, my dear readers, is one of the most challenging subjects to discuss. Why is it so challenging? I attended a conference once and the discussion came up regarding sexual perceptions in men versus women. We know that boys are reared differently than girls and sexual predilections are ingrained early in life. We also know that society regards male sexuality differently than female sexuality, and it is easy to get caught up in society's perception of how we should be. However, it wasn't until I attended a sexual health conference that I saw this set of pictures that really summed it up.

A Hot Mess

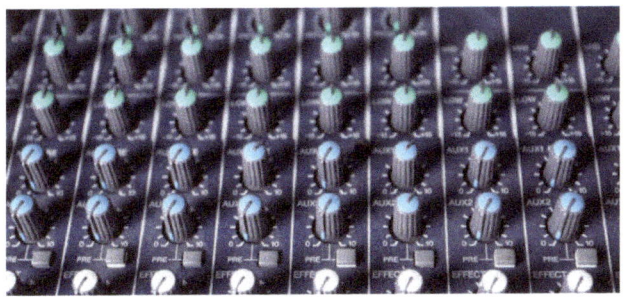

The sexual control knobs of women.

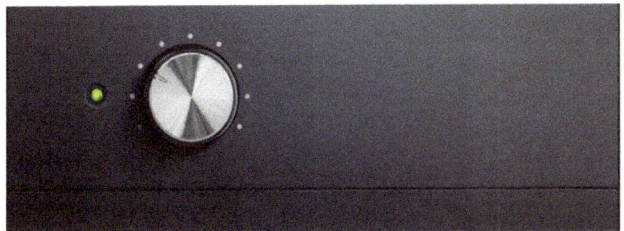

The sexual control knob of men.

Men and women are clearly wired differently. While men pretty much have one knob to turn them on sexually, women have many more knobs that make women much more complex. There are many cultural, emotional, spiritual, and just "life occurrences" that can influence women's moods and desires. Women are creatures of emotion and circumstance.

> *Did he take out the trash today or did I have to do it for the third week in a row?*
>
> *You did not get the promotion that you were hoping for and now you are really upset.*

You found a stack of nude photos in his drawer and you don't have a mole on that side of your butt.

All humans have deeply held personal factors that contribute to our feelings. Since there are so many influencers that contribute to the female libido, there is not one single solution for all women. Almost anything can affect the female sex drive.

Let us begin by defining the terms sexual desire and sexual health. Sexual desire is one's interest in sex and in being sexual. The three components of sexual desire are sexual drive, sexual attitude, and sexual motivation. Sexual health is defined as a state of physical, emotional, mental, and social well-being as it relates to sexuality.

Sexual Desire
Sexual drive, defined as the biological component of sexual desire, shows up as sexual thoughts, attraction to others, and the degree to which sexual activity is sought after. Genital arousal is included in this component. The sexual drive that each woman has is variable and is related to her menstrual cycle, daily activities, daily stressors, and overall health and well-being.

One's personal attitude regarding sex is the second component. A woman's attitude is influenced by numerous factors including her religious beliefs, her family's beliefs surrounding sex, her cultural beliefs, and even the media. The more positive or negative a woman's attitude is toward sex, the more positive or negative her attitude will be toward sexual desire.

The final and most complex component of sexual desire is motivation. This component includes a woman's willingness to be sexual with her partner, which is influenced by many factors. Since a woman's sexual desire is influenced by so many factors, it is not surprising that solutions to the problems are so varied. One of the most important factors to examine in sexual health is that not every problem or dysfunction is a problem for every woman or couple. For instance, a single woman with a decreased libido secondary to menopause may not care that she has a decreased sex drive. However, for a menopausal woman in a new sexual relationship with a younger partner, it can be a huge problem for her and her mate. Additionally, for a man on blood pressure medication with a blunted sexual appetite, his partner's vaginal dryness may not be a concern.

Decreased Libido

As hormone levels in the perimenopausal/menopausal woman decline, generally so does the libido. Minimal change occurs between the ages of forty-five and fifty-five, however, between ages fifty-five and sixty-five, there is a gradual and steady decline in libido. Although most women have a decline in sex drive during the transition, there are some who notice no significant change. Alternatively, a cadre of women feel liberated from the concern of getting pregnant and find an increase in their libido.

Although the big three—estrogen, progesterone, and testosterone—play a huge role in the menopausal transition, it is the hormone testosterone that appears to have the largest role in sex drive. Testosterone belongs to a group of hormones called androgens.

Testosterone? Yes, testosterone is not just for men. Women produce approximately one-tenth the amount of testosterone that men do. Testosterone, produced in the female ovaries and the adrenal glands, has its greatest decline at menopause such that a fifty-year-old woman makes about 50 percent of the hormone as her twenty-five-year-old counterpart. In addition to menopause, testosterone levels can decline during chemotherapy and other treatments.

Testosterone has many functions in men such as sperm production, building muscle mass, development of the sexual organs, fat distribution, and the production of red blood cells. In women, functions of testosterone include:

- Keeping the skin supple
- Assisting estrogen with its duties
- Building bone
- Creating a feeling of overall well-being and euphoria
- Maintaining libido
- Promoting high energy
- Minimizing depression

Mood Swings

There are notable signs and symptoms associated with mood swings during the transition. Irritability is common in many menopausal women who find themselves less tolerant and more easily provoked. Even the slightest little annoyance turns into a big production. Depression affects up to 20 percent of women while anxiety, worry, and panic attacks are common. Women tend to have more crying spells during the change.

The decline in estrogen during the transition can cause a decline in other hormones such as serotonin and norepinephrine. Serotonin and norepinephrine tend to be calming hormones, and with a reduction in them, there is an increase in anxiety. Women who seem to be the most plagued by mood swings are women with a history of PMS (premenstrual syndrome). The menopausal woman may find herself depressed about her symptoms, which can in turn increase the mood swings.

Hot Flashes (Vasomotor Symptoms)

"Doctor, why am I so hot when everyone else in the room is comfortable?"

The dreaded hot flash or hot flush. As an obstetrician/gynecologist, the hot flash is probably the most common symptom I hear about. The vasomotor symptom—or the hot flash—occurs in the majority of women. Upwards of 80 percent of women will experience hot flashes. What exactly is a hot flash and why do they occur? A hot flash is caused by an abrupt decline in the amount of estrogen in the body with a sudden increase in the body temperature. When estrogen levels decline, there is a surge of the hormone adrenaline that signals to the body it is time for "a fight or a flight." In other words, a hot flash is actually a protective mechanism to ready our bodies for defense or to run away from danger in the event that we are attacked. Other symptoms that can accompany hot flashes include heart palpitations, dizziness, warmth feelings, and a sense of dread that something ominous is going to occur. The face becomes flushed. The blood pressure and heart rate increase and blood vessels dilate. Women can begin to have vigorous sweating. Hot flashes are usually felt from the waist up and typically last about thirty seconds and rarely can last up to ten minutes. Hot flashes occur any time of the day, and when they occur while sleeping they are termed "night sweats."

Night sweats are hot flashes that occur while we are sleeping or attempting to sleep. They lead to the common symptom of insomnia, which can plague the menopausal woman. It becomes cyclical since the lack of sleep increases anxiety and irritability, which can further make the symptoms worse. No wonder you are having a bad day at work—you didn't sleep last night!

Vasomotor symptoms can last anywhere from six months to two years into the menopausal transition. They have been known to extend ten years into menopause. Women who tend to have hot flashes well into their menopause are women who are cigarette smokers or those with anxiety disorders. It is not uncommon for them to stop after a year or two and then restart later during the 'pause' years. African American and Hispanic American women tend to experience menopausal symptoms longer than women of other ethnicities.

THE URINARY SYSTEM

"I might as well buy stock in those diapers because I am buying them right and left."

The genitourinary system consists of the organs of both the reproductive system and the urinary system and since they are both derived from the same embryological tissue they are both affected by menopause.

Urinary Incontinence

The urinary system, consisting of the two kidneys that manufacture urine, two ureters carrying the urine to the bladder for storage and the urethra, which carries urine outside of the body are affected by menopause. Urinary incontinence, the involuntary loss of urine occurs in about 40 percent of perimenopausal and menopausal women making it commonplace. During the act of urinary incontinence urine is expelled from the bladder at an undesirable time. Our brains are involved in helping to control urinary leakage by telling us when it is culturally and socially appropriate to relieve ourselves.

The urethra as it carries urine from the bladder to outside the body is strongly influenced by the hormone estrogen.

During our younger years, the body's estrogen keeps the urethra pliable and flexible while the aging process causes it to lose tone and flexibility becoming stiff. As it stiffens, it is less capable of sealing off the urine and leakage happens. Pregnancy, childbirth and gravity also contribute to incontinence symptoms. The stiffer urethra is more susceptible to tears, which lead to an increase in bladder infections.

The three primary types of incontinence are stress, urge and mixed incontinence and as we age they become more common. During stress incontinence, the pressure in the abdomen is greater than the pressure in the urethra and simple everyday activities such as coughing, sneezing and laughing cause urinary leakage. Menopausal women can also experience urge incontinence or the overactive bladder. In urge incontinence before a woman has time to pull down her underwear she leaks urine secondary to contractions that are happening too soon. Other disease processes such as infection and disorders of the urinary system can cause incontinence. Mixed incontinence consists of stress incontinence, urge incontinence and the less common types of incontinence.

The aging bladder begins to lose its elasticity and volume holding capability. Additionally, pelvic floor muscles weaken with age, contributing to urinary leakage.

More often than not you will be glad you took the high road even if no one is there to watch.

CHAPTER 4

THE NERVOUS AND CARDIOVASCULAR SYSTEMS ON MENOPAUSE

"I came into this room to get something but I forgot what it was."

"My heart keeps fluttering and my primary care doctor has run every test and tells me there is nothing wrong with my heart."

THE NERVOUS SYSTEM

The central nervous system (CNS) consists of the brain and spinal cord and has a multitude of functions. The brain acts as the orchestrator of our involuntary and voluntary movements, the source of our thoughts, and the interpreter of our environment. It acts by receiving signals from the environment from sensory organs such as the eyes, ears, nose, tongue, and skin. The spinal cord acts as the communication conduit between the brain and the rest of the body, allowing messages to be sent and received. The remaining part of the nervous system, termed the peripheral nervous system, includes nerves outside the brain and spinal cord that allow for connecting the brain and spinal cord to the rest of the body.

Your high school best friend is turning fifty next week and she knows that you are the best strawberry cake baker east of the Mississippi. After all, you have been making a strawberry cake for her birthday for the past thirty years, and you can make the cake in your sleep. Well of course you agree that year thirty-one will be no different and you will be happy to make her cake. You want it to be fresh so you decide to wake up early the morning of the party to bake it.

As you look through your kitchen cabinet you don't see everything that you need for the cake. Well, at least, you don't think you do. Or maybe you do. You don't remember. You don't remember the necessary ingredients for the cake you've been baking for thirty years. After thirty years of making the same cake year after year, you cannot remember all the ingredients. What just happened? *Brain fog.*

The brain is the last frontier of the human body. This phenomenal organ weighing about three pounds is nothing short of a miracle. There has not been a computer made that could rival the human brain. The brain has the ability to communicate within itself and with other organs in the body. The sex steroid hormones estrogen and progesterone have a role in maintaining brain health. Estrogen and progesterone receptors are within the human brain, and when these hormone levels decrease, women can experience cognitive decline, depression, and mood swings—just to name a few. The perimenopausal and menopausal patient complains of depression. There are estrogen receptors located in the brain, thus there is a link between depression and decreased estrogen.

It is established that there are many estrogen receptors in the brain. What does that mean? It means that estrogen plays a huge role in the activities of our brain. With the declining estrogen levels during menopause, there will be some "senior moments." Estrogen affects other chemicals including serotonin and endorphins, resulting in an increase in emotional lability. Serotonin is one of the calming chemicals, so as it decreases there is an increase in anxiety and irritability. Anxiety and irritability can lead to more benign heart palpitations. Headaches tend to be more common during the menopausal transition.

Women during this time will find they may burst into tears while watching a simple commercial or may think the end of the world is near because they overcooked the Thanksgiving turkey. The women who seemed to be most bothered by the "brain on menopause" symptoms are those who were bothered by PMS symptoms including mood swings, depression, and anxiety. In fact, some patients report to me that they feel like they are PMSing all the time now. How do the brain symptoms associated with menopause differ from other mood swings? These complex changes tend to occur gradually. Menopausal women may find themselves having more trouble concentrating on the tasks at hand and often describe their symptoms as if they are walking around in a fog. The memory lapses may occur more frequently in menopause. We all have moments of forgetfulness in life. We may forget where we placed the car keys or not remember the last name of someone we went to school with. These moments are common and don't necessarily signal the beginning of dementia, although moments like these can be annoying and frustrating. It would be much more concerning if one did not remember what a car key was used for than where the car key is located.

THE CARDIOVASCULAR SYSTEM

"I didn't have high blood pressure until I went through the change."

The cardiovascular system (CVS) consisting of the heart, blood, blood components, and blood vessels functions as the transportation system of the body. This system functions to provide oxygen and nutrients to the body while carrying waste products out for removal.

As the heart ages, there are more things that can go wrong with it. Heart disease is the number one killer of women, with half of all deaths in women older than fifty being due to cardiovascular disease. These deaths are due primarily to strokes, high blood pressure (hypertension), and heart attack. Around the age of fifty, there is a substantial increase in the risk of heart disease so that at age sixty-five, a woman's chance of death from heart disease is the same as a man of that age. It is also well established that women who go through menopause prematurely have an increased risk of heart disease at the time of their premature menopause. As we age, there is the increased risk of the effects of simply living on the heart. Negative lifestyle habits such as cigarette smoking, sedentary living, and a high-fat diet contribute to the detrimental effects on the aging heart. Factors that contribute to heart disease include:

- Diabetes Mellitus
- Cigarette smoking
- Hypertension
- Obesity
- Sedentary lifestyle
- Strong family history of heart disease
- Elevated LDL (the undesirable cholesterol)
- Reduced HDL (the desirable cholesterol)

The hormone estrogen plays a role in the cardiovascular system. With the decline in estrogen, there is an increase in the accumulation of plaque in the blood vessels. This leads to an increase in the risk of strokes and heart attacks. The decline in estrogen can cause an increase in cholesterol, which can further increase the plaque in the blood vessels. Heart palpitations, heart racing, and heart fluttering are attributed to the hormonal changes and are usually harmless.

Barbara Ann Hannah, MD, MS, FACOG

"Be very careful who you disrespect, disregard, dismiss or dishonor in the flesh because you have no idea their rank in the spirit."

—UNKNOWN

CHAPTER 5

THE INTEGUMENTARY AND DIGESTIVE SYSTEMS ON MENOPAUSE

"My skin used to be so soft, but now it is scratchy and itches all the time."

THE INTEGUMENTARY SYSTEM

"I am not smiling, so why are those smile lines still there? It is not funny!"

The skin is the largest part of the body as well as the largest component of the integumentary system. We sometimes forget that the skin is an organ when in fact the skin is the largest organ in the body, weighing in at approximately ten pounds. Other parts of the integumentary system include the hair, nails, and accessory organs such as the sweat and sebaceous glands.

While the other body systems may bring about more heightened and noticeable changes, the menopausal changes in the integumentary system may take a while to notice. The menopausal woman notices the irregular periods, the hot flashes, and vaginal dryness, but the skin changes tend to be more gradual and subtle. Over time, the aging process causes the skin to become more brittle and to sag. Gravity weighs down all parts of the body, and skin changes are quite noticeable. Due to the lack of estrogen, the connective tissue fibers that help to create supple and pliant skin begin to deteriorate. Skin also loses its flexibility due to the decrease in the fatty layer under the skin. Blood vessels become more visible as the skin becomes thinner. Casual bruising happens more readily. During the menopausal years, hair loss is more common because estrogen and testosterone play a role in activating hair follicles. As hormone levels change, women observe less hair on their heads and more hair on their chins. Hair loss on the crown of the head, female pattern baldness, is an annoying symptom in some women.

Another change is the decrease in subcutaneous fat or fat located under the skin. This leads to an increase in wrinkles and a loss of flexibility. When you pull on the skin over your hand, it takes longer to get back to the place it once was! With the decrease in the fatty layer of the skin, the skin thins and blood vessels are more visible. The skin bruises more easily during this time, and its ability to regenerate itself diminishes. Dry and itchy skin is more of a problem for menopausal women due to a decrease in the oil production of the sebaceous glands. The thinning of the skin also leads to delayed wound healing and acne increases.

The ultraviolet light of the sun can destroy the collagen fibers leading to an acceleration of skin wrinkling. With time, the exposure of the skin to excessive sunlight contributes to skin cancer, especially in the fair-skinned population.

With the decline in hormone production, hair growth slows while hair loss increases. It is the change in testosterone that causes more hair loss by shrinking hair follicles, which in turn causes hair loss. In extreme cases, women experience more profound hair loss at the crown of the head and the sides. This is termed female pattern hair loss (FPHL) and does affect a cadre of women. FPHL occurs primarily with aging but can occur earlier being exacerbated by stress, medications, genetics, and diseases such as thyroid disease. Hair loss associated with such things as extreme scalp itching, red and dry scalp, pain and rapidly losing hair should be considered for professional evaluation. In these instances, the hair loss may be related to an underlying medical condition.

The changes in the integumentary system can certainly affect our self-image. The effects of constant muscle movement, sun exposure, generalized inflammation, hormonal changes, gravity, and certain medications contribute to these skin changes.

THE DIGESTIVE SYSTEM

"I have tried to eat more fruits and vegetables but I am still so backed up. It has been a week since I pooped."

"I cannot hold my farts. I was in a meeting last week and it just came out. Everybody tried to play it off but they knew it was me."

"I have been riding the bike every day for the past six months and I still cannot get rid of my stomach."

The components of the digestive system include the salivary glands, the mouth, the esophagus leading from the mouth to the stomach, the stomach, the small and large intestines, the rectum, and anus.

The GI (gastrointestinal) tract, or digestive system, has a myriad of functions. The organs of this system work together to not only digest food and provide it to the other parts of the body but also function as part of the immune system. During the perimenopausal and menopausal transitions, women begin to experience problems with their GI tract from incomplete digestion, which increases passing of gas and abdominal bloating, to constipation. Menopause also causes a decline in the good bacteria in the digestive system. These beneficial bacteria aid in the digestion of food, assist in nutrient absorption, and minimize the "bad" bacteria that can lead to malabsorption and flatulence.

Another potentially disturbing problem in the aging woman related to the decline in estrogen is the menopausal belly. Body fat is shifted to the midsection of the body especially to the sides and in the front. The increase in the hormone cortisol causes an increase in abdominal fat leading to more hypertension, diabetes, and heart disease.

*"When there is no enemy within you,
the enemy outside can do you no harm."*

—AFRICAN PROVERB

CHAPTER 6

THE RESPIRATORY AND MUSCULOSKELETAL SYSTEMS ON MENOPAUSE

"Why does this old volleyball injury hurt now when it didn't before?"

"I seem to be having a harder time catching my breath after even light exercise. I have always been fit."

THE RESPIRATORY SYSTEM
The respiratory system allows us to breathe by absorbing oxygen and eliminating waste in the form of carbon dioxide. The components of the respiratory system include the mouth, nose, sinuses, pharynx, trachea, bronchi, bronchial tubes, and the lungs. The accessory lung muscles also contribute to breathing.

The respiratory system efficiently works to pull in air from the environment via the nose and mouth, while the sinuses function to humidify the inhaled air. Air is then carried via the pharynx to the trachea down to the lungs where oxygen is exchanged and carried into the bloodstream.

There are changes in the pulmonary or respiratory system as we age. Menopausal women may notice that they are becoming short of breath easier than before. In menopausal women, the forced vital capacity and the forced expiratory volume change. The forced vital capacity is the measurement of the lung size while the forced expiratory volume is the amount of air that can be blown out in one second. So what does all that mean for the menopausal lady? These changes can cause an increase in shortness of breath and fatigue. Additionally, there is a reduction in the work capacity in the menopausal woman caused by these declines. Women who smoke cigarettes have an even sharper decline in respiratory function.

THE MUSCULOSKELETAL SYSTEM

Our skeletal system with its 206 bones is in a constant state of change and remodeling. The primary hormones affecting bone growth are growth hormones and the sex steroid hormones. The sex steroids—estrogen, progesterone, and testosterone—play a major role in the building and the breakdown of bone. Estrogen is vital in depositing the necessary calcium and magnesium needed to strengthen bone. Estrogen and testosterone promote the bone building activity of the osteoblastic cell.

The process of bone breakdown and bone remodeling is a dynamic and lifelong process. The skeletal system begins to form early in the uterus. During childhood, bones grow in length and thickness. Bone thickness, or bone density, reaches its peak around age thirty, after which there is bone loss. During our growth years, bone development is greater than bone resorption, and the formation of new bone is the primary process.

The decrease in estrogen, testosterone, and progesterone causes an increase in bone loss, termed osteoporosis. Osteoporosis is often confused with arthritis. Wherein arthritis is inflammation associated with joints, osteoporosis is a condition where there is thinning of the bones. There may or may not be pain associated with osteoporosis. When the osteoporosis is less severe, it is termed osteopenia. Factors that contribute to this disease process include genetics, personal health history, and lifestyle.

STAGES OF OSTEOPOROSIS

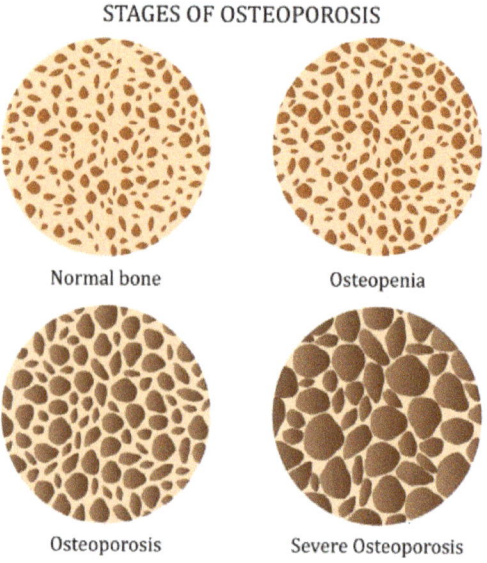

Normal bone

Osteopenia

Osteoporosis

Severe Osteoporosis

Osteopenia and osteoporosis are a debilitating cause for the well-known hip fractures that occur in menopausal women. In these conditions, bone density or thickness is reduced, which makes the bone more susceptible to fractures. Risk factors for osteoporosis include Caucasian race, thin body stature, and cigarette smoking. In osteopenia, bone density begins to decline but not enough to fracture—while in the more severe condition, osteoporosis, the weak and porous bone is more prone to fracture. This is why hip fractures in elderly women can be so debilitating.

Genetics and ethnicity play a role in the incidence of osteoporosis. Caucasian and Asian women have a higher rate of osteoporosis and osteopenia than women of African descent. While African American women have a 6 percent lifetime chance of developing osteoporosis, Asian and Caucasian women have a 14 percent lifetime risk of developing it.

A woman's personal history influences her likelihood of bone loss. For example, a woman's age at the time of menopause serves as a risk factor. The younger a woman is when she transitions, the longer her body is exposed to the declining estrogen levels and its consequences. Women who go through early menopause secondary to premature ovarian failure or surgical removal of the ovaries will be exposed longer to the declining estrogen levels. A woman's medicine history also plays a role. Corticosteroids, which are used to treat asthma, arthritis, and a number of other conditions, can weaken bone mass. Some thyroid medications and diuretics also hasten the effects of osteopenia and osteoporosis by reducing the amount of calcium in the body.

As we age, the hormonal changes decrease the amount of calcium and magnesium available for bone absorption. Both calcium and magnesium are needed for adequate bone strength. Estrogen functions to deposit these elements into the bone. With the declining estrogen levels, less calcium and magnesium are in the bloodstream and available for deposit into the bones.

Menopause can cause joint pain that can affect the shoulders, knees, elbows, neck, and hands known as "menopausal arthritis." Women may notice more aches and discomfort upon awakening that tend to resolve with movement. One of the reasons weight gain is more common during the menopausal years is that women tend to not exercise or be as active because of the pain. The decrease in estrogen causes an increase in joint inflammation, which in turn leads to reductions in mobility and flexibility.

> *"I would rather be hated for who I am than loved for who I am not."*
>
> —KURT COBAIN

CHAPTER 7

THE IMMUNE SYSTEM ON MENOPAUSE

I was just diagnosed with a chronic disease. It seems that all my troubles happened once my periods stopped."

"I have had this persistent vaginal discharge since menopause and my doctor keeps telling me that I don't have an infection. What is going on?"

The immune system is a large network of organs, cells, and chemicals that assists the body in fighting off infection. This system undergoes constant changes from birth throughout life. Newborns have no developed immune system. As they reach their pubertal years, the immune system completely matures. With the menopausal changes, the immune system undergoes many changes, collectively termed *immunosenescence* or the aging immune system.

The components of the immune system include white blood cells, proteins called antibodies, the lymphatic system, bone marrow, the spleen, the complement system, bone marrow, and the thymus gland. Without our immune system, we would not be able to fight off infection. One of the most fascinating aspects of the immune system is that it has a memory that allows it to remember the "invaders" and to quickly recognize them when they return and to attack them quickly. The lymphatic system as part of the immune system functions to fight off cancer cells and to manage the fluid levels in the body.

The aging of the immune system leads to an increase in inflammation and a decrease in the ability of the immune system to ward off infection. The increase in autoimmune disorders such as lupus, rheumatoid arthritis, inflammatory bowel disease, and multiple sclerosis is thought to be contributed to by the decrease in estrogen and progesterone. Women are known to have more autoimmune diseases than men, with 78 percent of autoimmune diseases occurring in females.

The decreasing estrogen levels contribute to the thinning of the vaginal epithelium, which in turn leads to an increase in vaginal infections in the menopausal woman. There is evidence that there is a spike in the cases of human papillomavirus in the menopausal woman, which is the virus that causes abnormal Pap smears and cervical cancer. Human immunodeficiency virus (HIV) levels have been shown to increase in the menopausal patient, which is thought to be due to the decrease in the protective killer cells of the immune system. Cortisol, a stress hormone produced by the adrenal glands, increases in menopause, which in turn diminishes the capabilities of the immune system. The process of menopause with its associated symptoms of weight gain, memory loss, mood swings, and decreased libido is a stressful time for many women. This increase in the stress of menopause causes an increase in cortisol levels, further reducing the efficacy of the immune system.

All parts of the immune system are affected including the thymus gland, which is located behind the breastbone or sternum. This gland, which functions to produce protective T-cells, shrinks as we age while making fewer T-cells. The decrease in T-cells makes the menopausal woman more susceptible to chronic conditions such as cancer and rheumatoid arthritis.

Some of the menopausal symptoms actually weaken the immune system. The sleep deprivation associated with menopause weakens the immune system and since sleep is such a vital contributor to a healthy immune system, the immune system suffers. Additionally, vaginal dryness can cause a decrease in sexual activity, and it is well known that sexual activity heightens the immune response.

> *"Be careful not to use the eyes of others to see yourself."*

CHAPTER 8

TREATMENT OF MENOPAUSAL SYMPTOMS, PART I

"How am I going to get through menopause? Is there something out there that can help me?"

In the United States, the life expectancy for men is 75.1 years while the life expectancy for women is 80.5 years. With the average age of menopause being 52.4 years, that means the average woman can expect to live within her menopausal years for almost thirty years.

Since we are only given so much time on this earth, then why not make the most of it? Father Time waits for no one and the minutes of the day tick by for all of us at the same rate. Our perception of time, however, is different. When we were children, it seemed forever for our birthdays and holidays to roll around. Growing up I could not understand my parents saying how fast time was passing because as a child I didn't see it that way. With age, we cannot seem to catch up to time and it seems to fly by. How often do we find ourselves commenting on how time flies and wishing that we had more time in the day? I have often wondered why it seems to pass quickly as we age. Perhaps it is because we have more to do with our time. Yes, our time. We all are allocated a specific amount of time in which to live this life. The price we pay for living this life is aging because as time passes so does our chronological clock. It is inevitable. My mother used to say regarding the aging process, "We are either old or cold." I believe that I am correct in saying that most of us would rather be old.

The aging woman will go through the change. As aging is inevitable, so is menopause. Since turning back the hand of time is not an option, we must think of ways to make our menopausal years happy, productive, and dynamic. It does us no good to continually deny the process of the change. There may be moments that we wish we could still run our high school 220 in twenty-two seconds or wish we could wear the bikini that our college boyfriend gave us while all the time turning heads. The occasional nostalgic thoughts are normal, but to dwell on the past is not useful. How long are we going to be wistful? Hopefully not long because we want to get on living our best lives.

I believe that the initial step in the treatment of the menopausal woman is her acceptance of the aging process—the acceptance of herself. Once we have accepted the changes, it is important to educate ourselves on how to make this time the best that we can. I encourage you to be cognizant of your own body, your mind, and your spirit. Know yourself. Honor yourself. Be patient with yourself. Love yourself. Above all, be good to yourself because there is only one you and you have all that you need to be the best person that you can be. Remember your uniqueness and that you are worth the effort it takes to manage this time in your life.

Are you familiar with that menopausal woman who is so comfortable in her own skin and exudes confidence in her daily walk? She has traded her youthful years for wisdom and security. She embraces who she is and the changes in her life. She is being uniquely herself. You want to be in her presence because she makes you feel good about who you are. You want to be like her! Well, you can be with some fine tuning and lifestyle and mindset changes. I want you to live *your* best menopausal life. I want you to get your sexy back!

The Dry Vagina

> *"Last night, Nick was in tears because I was hurting so much. There was blood on our sheets afterwards. What can you do to help me?"*

If I had to select the most worrisome and emotionally concerning symptom of menopause, it would be the vaginal dryness that I hear about from most of my sexually active patients. This dryness or atrophic vaginitis is due to the decrease in the hormone estrogen leading to painful sexual intercourse. Importantly, once the process of vulvovaginal atrophy begins, it will continue to worsen unless treated. Ironically, one of the best ways to maintain a healthy vagina is to use it! Regular sexual activity with or without a partner increases the blood flow and elasticity of the vagina. Since none of us like to be in pain, the next question is, "how can I have sex if it is so painful?"

There are numerous over-the-counter, nonhormonal preparations that can be helpful. These products are classified as either moisturizers or lubricants. Moisturizers can be vaginally inserted every few days to add hydration to the vagina. I recommend that even women who are not sexually active utilize a moisturizer because a hydrated vagina is a healthier vagina.

Moisturizers adhere to the vaginal epithelium and cause a thin moist film to appear. The vagina will then absorb the amount of product needed and the rest will be excreted. Since these products are best used every few days they can also help to restore normal vaginal pH. Many vaginal moisturizers are on the market, and I advise women to research their options to determine what is best for them.

While moisturizers are added to the vaginal epithelium on a regular basis, vaginal lubricants are applied to the sexual organs at the time of sexual activity with the intent of relieving sexual discomfort and increasing pleasure. They have a viscous consistency mimicking that of the body's natural secretions. Lubricants can be water, oil, or silicone based. Water-based lubricants are easy to use, wash off readily, and are compatible with latex condoms. They can dry up quickly, requiring more product to be used.

Oil-based lubricants include vegetable, nut, coconut, and almond oils. The nut-based oils tend to be the most natural and cause minimal irritation if they are washed off properly. If not washed off properly, oil-based lubricants can cause infections. Also, they are not compatible with latex condoms causing breakdown of the condom. The silicone lubricant lasts longer than the water-based lubricant and can safely be used with latex condoms. They can be difficult to rinse off, leading to more vaginal irritation, but because they last longer, they can be used in smaller quantities than the water-based ones. Like the vaginal moisturizer, I encourage women to find the lubricant that works best for them. While the over-the-counter products work well for some patients, some women need prescription-strength treatment. In those cases, I will consider vaginal estrogen.

Low-dose vaginal estrogen is appropriate for a select group of women and helps to relieve vaginal dryness. Not all women are candidates for this type of treatment, so your provider input and a prescription are required. Vaginal estrogen serves to minimize the dryness and it relieves painful intercourse known as dyspareunia. Additionally, some of the urinary symptoms encountered in menopausal women can be reduced with vaginal estrogen. These low-dose products are effective in treating the atrophic vaginitis, and because these products are applied directly into the vagina, there is less systemic absorption, which lessens the body's exposure to the additional estrogen.

Vaginal estrogen comes in several formulations, which include creams, suppositories, rings, and tablets. The products are directly inserted into the vagina, and I recommend insertion initially at bedtime for two weeks followed by twice per week thereafter. Of note, once use of the product is stopped, the atrophic vaginitis will recur. Some preparations work better for some women than others, but most research shows equal efficacy. There is also a daily pill that can be used to minimize vaginal dryness and make intercourse more comfortable. Patients with breast cancer or who are at increased risk of developing it are cautioned about taking this pill. While vaginal estrogen can be a wonder drug for some women, it is not recommended for all women. Those women with a history of breast cancer and/or blood clots in the deep vessels of the body should speak with their medical provider regarding estrogen usage.

There is another pill option that is not an estrogen that can be used to help with vaginal dryness. This along with a DHEA steroid hormone can be used to minimize vaginal dryness. Nonmedical options are also available for the woman with vaginal dryness. There are carbon dioxide vaginal laser treatments aimed at treating the vaginal epithelium. These treatments work by creating microscopic, non-painful tears that will heal over time. This healed vaginal tissue is stronger, healthier, and has a heightened blood supply. These procedures are not covered by insurance. These products and treatments can help the menopausal woman get her groove back.

THE HOT FLASH (VASOMOTOR SYMPTOM)

"Is anyone else in here hot?"

The vasomotor symptom, or hot flash, occurs when blood vessels dilate, heat is given off, and the body temperature rises. These changes occur as a result of a decline in estrogen and changes in testosterone and cortisol. With the hot flash, dizziness, redness, perspiration, heart palpitations, and facial flushing can occur.

The triggers of the hot flash vary from patient to patient, but there are some triggers that seem to be relatively common. The food we consume can dilate or narrow blood vessels. Spicy foods such as chili peppers and cayenne, for example, have a heat-producing ingredient in them called capsaicin. Capsaicin dilates blood vessels, which in turn can cause hot flashes. Consuming alcohol can also trigger hot flashes by causing blood vessels to dilate, which causes a sensation of warmth. This is why the skin flushes when drinking a glass of wine. Consumables containing caffeine can also be a trigger because caffeine affects the blood vessels.

There are some foods that can help relieve hot flashes and are good for us as well. These foods contain a compound called phytoestrogens. Phytoestrogens are compounds that are derived from plants and can decrease hot flashes by mimicking the body's natural estrogen. Foods that are high in phytoestrogens include broccoli, blueberries, carrots, oranges, peas, beans, tea, and avocado. Phytoestrogens are manufactured in a synthetic pill form, however, I prefer the natural fruits and vegetables. For women with a history of breast cancer, please consult your medical provider regarding phytoestrogen consumption.

Excessive heat can also cause hot flashes. Hot weather or excessive clothing can be triggers because they cause the skin temperature to increase, therefore aggravating hot flashes. Dressing in layers can be beneficial since layers can be removed if a woman gets uncomfortable. Breathable fabric like cotton will be more comfortable than nylon or spandex.

Lastly, women who smoke cigarettes often experience more hot flashes. No matter the body system, there is nothing healthy about smoking—and that includes its effects on menopause. Cigarette smoking makes hot flashes worse by increasing the frequency and severity of them. Additionally, women who smoke cigarettes enter menopause one to two years sooner than their nonsmoking counterparts.

I encourage women to maintain a diet rich in fruits and vegetables. Not only does a healthy diet including fruits and vegetables help to decrease hot flashes, but it provides weight control and decreases the occurrence of some chronic illnesses such as heart disease and cancer. Since hot flashes can increase stress levels, deep breathing techniques can be beneficial by decreasing anxiety. Although exercise can sometimes initiate a hot flash, it is a wonderful way to feel better overall and can help to minimize the frequency of hot flashes. In combination with other techniques to manage hot flash symptoms, some women choose to carry a portable fan.

URINARY INCONTINENCE

"When I have to go, I have to go!"

Urinary incontinence, defined as the loss of bladder control, can be an embarrassing problem. Upwards of 40 percent of women are plagued with this concern. For some menopausal women, the leakage is mild, while others have more severe bladder control issues. With the passage of time, the pelvic floor weakens due to childbirth, gravity, excessive straining, and time. This weakening of the pelvic floor contributes to incontinence.

Prior to treating urinary incontinence, a thorough history and physical should be performed. A urinalysis is done to identify signs of infection as well as detect numerous disease processes such as diabetes, dehydration, and kidney disease. Included in the history is the timeframe of when the symptoms began, the frequency of the incontinence, and other medical conditions.

In a small cadre of women with minimal symptoms, simple bladder retraining to hold urine a bit longer is helpful. By incrementally holding the urine longer, the bladder becomes stronger. Kegel exercises help to strengthen the pelvic floor muscles by strengthening the pubococcygeus muscle, which in turn helps to control the flow of urine. In order to perform Kegels, simply stop the flow of urine midstream by squeezing the muscle. Squeeze that same muscle for three seconds and then release and allow urine to flow. This repetitive squeeze and release helps to strengthen the pubococcygeus muscle while helping to reduce the flow of unwanted urine. Kegel exercises can be done any time of the day or night. If you are unsure if you are performing the exercise properly, don't be embarrassed to seek help from your provider.

If behavioral techniques are ineffective, there is medical therapy to treat the overactive bladder or urge incontinence. Since the bladder and the vagina are derived from the same embryological tissue, vaginal estrogen in addition to helping vaginal dryness can help with bladder incontinence. By simply inserting vaginal estrogen into the vagina, the bladder symptoms can improve. Medical therapy in pill form relaxes the bladder and counteracts the contractions that are causing urinary leakage. Common side effects of these medications include dry mouth, dry eyes, and constipation. Sipping on water and sugar-free candy can help relieve the dry mouth while eye drops can help to relieve the dry eyes. I recommend fiber rich diets, stool softeners, and bulk laxatives to help decrease the side effects of the medications.

Other techniques to assist with urinary incontinence include bladder injections and nerve stimulation. A protein injected directly into the bladder has been used to treat severe incontinence and its beneficial effects can last for up to one year. Repeat injections are often required. Bladder infections are associated with this treatment.

Another technique to minimize incontinence is nerve stimulation where a thin wire or needle is placed in the lower back or the ankle and delivers impulses to the urinary bladder. The sacral nerve, located in the lower back, can be manipulated by placing a device in the back that can control the impulses from the bladder to the brain. This device acts like a pacemaker to block the messages to the brain. The end result is the reduction in incontinence episodes.

Bulking agents can be injected into the urethra and increase the size of the urethra allowing the urethra to remain closed until urination is desired. This procedure requires repeat injections.

Surgical procedures to relieve urinary incontinence include suspensions, slings, and mesh. The suspension procedure is done to lift the bladder and reattach it in a different location. During a sling procedure, a device is placed around the bladder neck to provide support and prevent leakage. Vaginal mesh surgery has fallen out of favor due to complications that have arisen such as mesh erosion. In this procedure, a piece of tape is inserted behind the urethra to elevate it.

A device that can help to alleviate incontinence by delivering electromagnetic pulses to the pelvic floor is now on the market. This FDA-approved device functions to deliver thousands of Kegel exercises to the pelvic floor while the patient is sitting fully clothed. This procedure is not covered by insurance.

Multiple treatment options are available for the common problem of urinary incontinence. There is no need for the dynamic menopausal woman to suffer from incontinence. I encourage you to talk with your healthcare provider to determine the best option(s) for you.

DECREASED SEX DRIVE

"I told Betty not to come over last night. I was not in the mood."

Menopause commonly causes a decrease in the libido. Multiple factors are causative including the decrease in hormones, weight gain, change of body perception and fatigue. I often hear about the changes in sexual health during menopause. I recommend attempting to identify the problem because different problems have different solutions. Since so many factors contribute to our sexual health, there is not one solution. Women are complex beings and so many factors contribute to our sexual health. These include our physical changes, cultural and religious background, self-image, and lifestyle to name a few.

Hypoactive sexuality is a good time to reevaluate the relationship. Be transparent about your feelings and expect your partner to be the same. It is not fair of us to expect our partners to be mind-readers. They may not understand all that we are feeling so it is our responsibility to educate them. Participating in other sensual and intimate activities together such as bathing, massaging, or watching a sexy movie can be exciting. Try to keep the focus on intimacy and less on the act of intercourse. As previously mentioned, what may be a problem in one relationship may not necessarily be a problem in another. A couple with one partner on blood pressure medication and the other on chemotherapy may not have a sexual problem while the menopausal woman and her new younger lover may have a big problem.

Self-pleasure during menopause can be beneficial. One of the benefits of masturbation is that it increases the immune system, which has benefits for the menopausal woman.

Sexual issues are contributed to by the decrease in libido, vaginal dryness, arousal issues, painful sex, and orgasm problems. Decreased libido can be addressed with sexual counseling. Sexual counseling can be helpful, and in order for it to be helpful, it is important to be transparent with the counselor. Certain medications such as antidepressants and high blood pressure medications can decrease the libido. I urge you to notify your medical provider to review your medications. I use low-dose testosterone in some of my patients, which helps to increase libido.

Yoga along with regular exercise can be a boost for sexual health by both increasing the blood flow to the vital organs and causing a relaxing and calming effect. Both yoga and exercise increase the release of endorphins, which have a calming effect and trigger positive emotions. I recommend thirty minutes of exercise most days of the week. Prior to any exercise program, be sure to get the blessings of your medical provider.

There is a medication that, when applied to the clitoris, can increase blood flow. This medication has had a modest effect in my menopausal patients. Additionally, there is clitoral surgery that reduces the size of the prepuce or clitoral hood. This technique may allow for more stimulation during intercourse. I would caution my menopausal women about this technique since the clitoris already becomes smaller in menopause. The use of vibrators can help some women.

Minimizing alcohol intake can help counteract hypoactive sexuality, since multiple glasses of alcohol can diminish the libido. Avoiding heavy meals prior to sex can also help.

When it comes to sexual concerns, there is no "one size fits all." What works for one woman and her partner may not work for another. There is no "normal" frequency for intercourse, which is variable from woman to woman. Transparency in communication is vital. Human beings are complex creatures, and this is a complex topic. Most women want to have a certain level of sexual desire and to have that desire satisfied. As our bodies age, we need to rethink what our bodies look like to us. In the past, areas that used to be tight and supple now begin to droop and sag and we want to learn to appreciate the new normal. Our body image plays a huge role in how we view our sexuality. The more we appreciate our body and the more confidence we have in ourselves, the more our partner will too. Creativity and variety also help to enhance our sex lives. Routine is the enemy of excitement so it may be worthwhile to plan a trip or try a new location. A different environment can be sexually appealing. This is your sex life and you only get one. Don't be afraid to be true to yourself.

"We are either old or cold."

—ELIZABETH C. HANNAH

CHAPTER 9

TREATMENT OF MENOPAUSAL SYMPTOMS, PART II

"I was given this big project at work and I kept having to review it over and over again to get it right."

BRAIN FOG

Menopause can bring about a reduction in memory, concentration, and cognition. Upwards of 50 percent of women experience these changes. These changes thought to be due to the hormonal decline become more noticeable with aging.

When it comes to dealing with the "brain on menopause," I recommend that women first realize that this is a normal occurrence and they are not going crazy. One of my recommendations is to attempt to minimize stress. Participating in relaxing activities, such as yoga and deep breathing exercises, can help increase mental concentration and reduce anxiety, stress, and depression. Adequate and frequent exercise causes an increase in brain oxygenation, leading to improved moods and less anxiety. The type of aerobic exercise that you choose to do is not as important as doing it on a frequent and consistent basis. The key is to find activities that you enjoy doing four to five times a week and to do them for thirty minutes per day.

The unhealthy habit of smoking cigarettes exacerbates menopausal symptoms by diminishing the amount of oxygen to the brain. For the woman who smokes cigarettes, there are numerous anti-smoking aids on the market. Even if you have attempted to stop smoking and have not been successful or have picked up the habit again, try again. In fact, don't quit quitting. The next time you try may be the successful one.

The internet is inundated with brain games and mind activities. I encourage you to participate in brain games to keep the brain exercised and the mind sharp. Involve yourself in stimulating activities such as visits to the museum, reading books, and stimulating conversations. One of the keys to minimizing the effects of the brain on menopause is to keep the brain active!

INSOMNIA

"Sometimes I am able to fall asleep but I keep waking up in the middle of the night."

The lack of sleep associated with menopause is very common. At least 50 percent of my patients say that insomnia is one of their biggest problems. Sleep disturbances include trouble falling asleep, staying asleep, and unintentional awakening. There are multiple reasons for menopausal sleep disturbances. The decrease in estrogen and progesterone during this time period affects the brain. The hot flashes and night sweats as a result of estrogen reduction interrupt sleep. With the sleep disturbances there is an increase in mood swings and irritability, which can further worsen the insomnia, becoming a vicious cycle. In addition to the decrease in hormones, insomnia is worsened by the increase in bathroom frequency during the night, termed nocturia. Arthritis is more common in the menopausal years, and these aches and pains can keep women awake. The sleep hormone melatonin decreases with age, further contributing to the sleep disturbances. Once thought to be a disease of men, sleep apnea has been found to affect women too, especially during the perimenopause/menopause transition. Because the causes of insomnia can be varied, I recommend that patients try to target the primary reason(s) for their sleep disturbances. Some helpful hints to combat sleep disturbances include:

- Regularly scheduled sleep: going to bed and awaking around the same time
- Minimize napping close to bedtime
- Minimize excess stimuli before bed including television, computer, or cell phone usage
- Avoidance of exercise close to bedtime
- Minimize large meals before bedtime
- Minimize caffeine before bedtime

Regular exercise and yoga have a calming effect on the body and enhance sleep. I recommend not exercising too close to bedtime, which can be a stimulant and prevent adequate sleep. Menopausal women should aim for seven to eight hours of quality sleep per night. Attempting to maintain a regular sleep schedule is helpful. Keeping your bedroom temperature around sixty-five degrees is comfortable for most. Attempt to limit day time napping to no more than twenty minutes since this can interfere with getting adequate sleep.

I do recommend melatonin. I find that it can be helpful in relieving insomnia. Patients tend to fall asleep sooner with melatonin and get a better night's sleep. Additionally, it tends not to be as addictive as other sleep aids. The most common side effects of melatonin are headache, dizziness, drowsiness, and nausea. I recommend that caution be taken if driving or machine operation occurs within five hours of taking it.

ARTHRITIS

"My bones ache. I believe that I have had arthritis before the change but it is worse now. I am so busy that I cannot always get an exercise routine in my day. I do feel better when I exercise."

Estrogen helps to maintain joint flexibility and mobility. As we age, the decline in estrogen affects our joints. There is decreased flexibility, decreased mobility, and increased joint pain. Arthritis is more common in menopause. Arthritis is inflammation of joints that leads to pain and stiffness.

Maintaining a healthy weight and exercise can reduce arthritis symptoms. Also eating a balanced diet full of fruits and vegetables is beneficial by providing antioxidants that reduce inflammation. The addition of beans and nuts to the diet provide nutrients such as calcium and magnesium, which are important for healthy joints and bones. Vitamin supplements can be useful since acquiring adequate vitamins in our food can be challenging. Adequate water intake decreases joint inflammation by increasing joint lubrication. The daily amount of water intake should be half of your body weight in ounces such that a 150 lb. woman should drink 75 ounces of water per day.

Avoid exercises that put undue strain on the joints such as hard surface exercises. Swimming and bicycling are good exercises during menopause since they don't cause undue strain on the joints.

Other therapies for menopausal arthritis include acupuncture and hydrotherapy. Hydrotherapy involves exercises performed in a warm water pool and can increase range of motion and strength. Some women are finding that acupuncture can help to relieve joint pain and other menopausal symptoms. Nonsteroidal medications and steroid injections can be beneficial in helping to alleviate arthritis symptoms.

OSTEOPOROSIS

"My aunt Ruth just turned seventy-five and she has that hump in her back. Will I get that?"

Osteoporosis, the severe thinning of bones, can be debilitating for the postmenopausal woman. With the thinning of bones, there is an increased risk of fracture even without a fall. The recommended test for the evaluation of bone density is the DEXA (dual energy X-ray absorptiometry) scan. The DEXA scan is a high-energy X-ray that measures bone mineral density as well as bone loss. It is a safe and convenient test with a low level of radiation. I recommend this testing begin at age sixty-five or sooner in those patients with risk factors.

I prefer to treat bone health before osteopenia or osteoporosis becomes an issue. Debilitating consequences can occur from a fall or injury. Maintaining adequate calcium and vitamin D levels are important. I recommend that postmenopausal women ingest at least 1,200 milligrams of calcium per day. Good sources of calcium include low-fat dairy products, dark green leafy vegetables, tofu, and orange juice. In order for calcium to be properly absorbed, vitamin D is necessary. I recommend 800 international units of vitamin D per day in the average woman. More may be needed if there is a significant deficiency. Sunlight is a good source of vitamin D along with liver, eggs, sardines, and red meats.

Both calcium and vitamin D can be found in the diet, however, supplements are often necessary.

Having thyroid disease can exacerbate bone loss. It is important to maintain normal thyroid health and to correct overactive (hyperthyroidism) and underactive (hypothyroidism) thyroid conditions.

For women who have had bariatric surgery, it is necessary to add additional supplements since nutrient absorption can be compromised after the surgery.

Exercise is very important in combating and preventing osteoporosis and osteopenia. Exercise promotes continuous bone building and breakdown, leading to healthier bones. Those individuals with a sedentary lifestyle have more issues with bone loss. Cessation of cigarette smoking will help to slow the process of bone loss.

SKIN, HAIR, AND NAILS

"Oh, how I wish I had not laid out so much in the sun during my twenties."

Aging skin needs more moisture. Formulations that hydrate the skin tend to be better than foam or gel cleansers, which can have a drying effect. Adding moisturizers while the skin is still wet can help to seal in the moisture. Moisturizers with an SPF of thirty or higher can be helpful. Be cognizant of the billion-dollar skin care industry. There are more products on the market than you can shake a stick at. Some of them are worth your money and others are not. If necessary, contact your dermatologist with questions.

Adequate nutrition and water intake are important. Foods that are high in antioxidants help to increase collagen, which helps to maintain skin's suppleness. Soy-based products may also help improve skin quality. Adequate hydration leads to plumper, more youthful-appearing skin. What you put into your body is just as important as how you move it. Exercise increases blood circulation, which helps to slow the aging process. The skin that is exercised tends to look brighter and more radiant.

In addition to healthy internal factors, external factors will also play a role. Excess sun exposure causes a premature decline in the collagen and elastin fibers, leading to an increase in skin damage along with an increased risk of skin cancer. Smoking cigarettes ages the skin, and smokers tend to have thinner skin than nonsmokers, which leads to an increase in wrinkles.

Most times hair loss in menopausal women is not related to an underlying condition. A diet rich in fiber and adequate vitamin intake can help to reduce the effects of hair loss in menopause. Diets high in vitamins A and C reduce hair loss by promoting hair growth. Vitamin C, found in some hair products, helps to aid in the hair's ability to absorb moisture. It also acts as an antioxidant to reduce hair damage. Vitamin B5, pantothenic acid, promotes hair growth by stimulating hair follicles. This vitamin can be found in eggs, fish, sweet potatoes, and tomatoes.

Iron and vitamin B12 in the diet can also help aid hair growth. Iron increases blood flow to the hair follicles while vitamin B12 specifically increases red blood cell delivery of oxygen to the hair follicle stimulating follicular growth. Zinc supplements can aid in the process by maintaining a balance of protein in the hair follicle necessary for growth.

Hair loss unrelated to an underlying condition can be managed with medications. Initially introduced as a treatment for high blood pressure, this medication was noted to cause an increase in overall body hair growth. Since then, medication has been approved to treat hair loss. It is applied directly to the scalp and massaged in. One of the side effects of this medication is scalp irritation. Since testosterone changes contribute to hair loss, anti-testosterone medications have been used to treat hair loss. These medications should be discussed with your provider.

The decrease in water and diminished hormones affect nails, making them more brittle and leading to easier cracking. Since nails are part of the integumentary system, I recommend the same diet rich in fiber, vitamins, and minerals that can help hair growth. Adequate water intake is important for maintaining nail integrity. Wearing gloves while performing household tasks can be helpful along with a good hand moisturizer.

"And the day came when the pain associated with remaining tight in the bud became greater than the pain it took to blossom."

—ANIAS NIN

CHAPTER 10

NUTRITION, EXERCISE, AND LIFESTYLE CHANGES IN MENOPAUSE

"I find that I feel so much better when I exercise. How much exercise do I really need?"

We live in a society that is enamored with the quick fix. We want a pill to fix this and a pill to fix that, and although medications certainly have a place in our lives, we often forget that food is medicine. Before we had medicine, many of our ancestors learned of the medicinal qualities of certain foods and utilized them to treat ailments. Times have changed and we have become more sophisticated, however, I believe that our bodies have been endowed with a certain inherent ability to heal themselves. We also know that foods have healing properties, and specific lifestyle patterns are associated with more optimal health. There are unique challenges associated with menopause, but with some extra effort, women in this transition can live their best lives.

We are aware that there is an increase in certain medical conditions as we age. As our hormone levels decrease and menopausal symptoms increase, the body's metabolism slows. Keeping the weight off is much more difficult. On average, caloric intake for the dynamic menopausal woman should be between 1,500 and 2,000 calories per day. The appropriate amount of caloric intake is related to height, weight, and activity level. We also know that a healthy diet, exercise, and lifestyle changes can help improve the quality of life, reduce some of the risks associated with diseases, and provide more energy. Healthy eating habits help by reducing chronic illnesses. A balanced and nutritious diet can also reduce some of the troubling symptoms associated with menopause.

Food is fuel and food is medicine. Although we eat for a variety of reasons, the primary reason is to provide fuel for our bodies. The right combination of food should include the macronutrients: carbohydrates, protein, and fat. Approximately 50 percent of our diet should include carbohydrates, 20 percent proteins, and 30 percent fats. Proteins, carbohydrates, and fats collectively work together for optimal health, and the right combination throughout the day will provide adequate energy for your daily activities.

BASIC FOOD GUIDELINES FOR MENOPAUSE AND PERIMENOPAUSE

Fifty percent of our diet should be composed of carbohydrates. These include foods like bread, fruits, vegetables, pasta, and cereals. To make the most of carbohydrate intake, menopausal women should aim for foods high in fiber, including the whole grains, fruits, and vegetables. Foods that are high in fiber are digested more slowly, so they will provide sustained energy throughout the day. Fresh foods are best when available, as they will provide the body with more nutrients than canned or processed foods. It should be noted that the recommended daily intake of fiber is twenty-one grams after the age of fifty, which is a decrease from the recommendation of twenty-five grams for younger women. However, since most people don't get enough fiber in their diet, aiming to consume foods high in fiber will certainly not hurt when a woman has reached her menopausal years.

Thirty percent of the diet should consist of fats. Fats provide more energy than proteins and carbohydrates but also contain more calories, which leads to greater weight gain. Saturated fats should make up 7 to 8 percent of your total daily calories and include those found in cheese, ice cream, whole milk, and fatty meats. Saturated fats will increase cholesterol levels. Be aware of the trans fat, which is found in fried foods, baked goods, and some margarines. These too elevate cholesterol levels as well as the risk for heart disease. The polyunsaturated and monounsaturated fats found in oils such as corn oil, safflower oil, olive oil, and peanut oil are preferred to the saturated and trans fats for reducing heart disease and some cancers.

Lastly, 20 percent of the diet should consist of protein. Protein is responsible for building and repairing tissue. Fish, lean meats, eggs, peas, and beans are high in protein.

The macronutrients aren't the only important components of a healthy diet. Vitamins, minerals, and antioxidants are crucial to a balanced diet. Calcium, vitamin D, and magnesium are necessary vitamins and minerals to create a balanced diet and a happy menopausal woman. Menopausal women need between 1,200 and 1,500 milligrams of calcium daily, so consuming foods like green leafy vegetables, dairy products, juices, salmon and sardines will help meet that quota. Calcium is crucial to bone development and menopausal women are at risk for bone loss. Vitamin D is necessary for the absorption of calcium. Before age seventy, 600 international units (IUs) of vitamin D are required, while after age seventy, that recommendation increases to 800 IUs. Magnesium is necessary to regulate a variety of functions, and a body low in magnesium will easily get muscle cramps, headaches, mood swings, and disrupted sleep.

Antioxidants are chemicals that help to reduce free radicalization in the body. Free radicals are chemicals that promote or enhance toxic reactions, so it is wise to eliminate them when we can. As the body ages, the antioxidant levels decline, leaving the body susceptible to medical issues such as heart disease and osteoporosis. Foods that are high in antioxidants are the colorful fruits and vegetables such as carrots, grapes, berries, and broccoli. Consuming more of these during menopause is recommended.

With the decline in estrogen, adding phytoestrogens to your meal plan is a good idea. Phytoestrogens are plant-based estrogens, which have been found to reduce cholesterol and support the immune system. Examples of these are found in tofu, soy yogurt, and other soy products. In fact, soy phytoestrogens are sometimes used as an alternative to hormone replacement therapy for the treatment of menopausal symptoms! Women who cannot take estrogens should speak with their providers before consuming additional phytoestrogens.

Adequate hydration is important in the menopausal years. Our bodies are 70 percent water and we constantly lose water through urination, perspiration, and breathing. It is recommended that we drink one-half of our body weight in ounces per day. A woman weighing 200 pounds therefore should drink 100 ounces of water daily. Many of the menopausal issues such as dry itchy skin, joint inflammation, memory loss, headaches, fatigue, and more can simply be helped by consuming more water!

Now that we've discussed what to include in a healthy diet for a menopausal woman, let's discuss what to minimize. First is alcohol consumption. A moderate amount of alcohol may be beneficial in minimizing heart disease and increasing HDL cholesterol, the good cholesterol. The recommendation is not to exceed two glasses of wine per day. Additionally, alcohol can intensify hot flashes, so be sure to drink water when consuming alcohol as well.

Caffeine can increase hot flashes while decreasing blood calcium. The decrease in blood calcium has the potential of increasing osteoporosis. Similarly, diets high in salt have been linked to a decrease in bone density as well as an increase in high blood pressure. I also encourage women to decrease excessive sugar since it has been linked to heart disease and cancer. While it may be nice to have the "sugar high," it only gives a quick boost of energy followed by a huge letdown. It is far better to indulge in the complex carbohydrates for more sustained energy.

EXERCISE GUIDELINES FOR THE MENOPAUSAL WOMAN

Before beginning any exercise regimen, consulting a medical provider is recommended. That being said, if a woman has not exercised much before menopause, now is a great time to start! Exercise for menopausal women has a myriad of benefits including preventing weight gain, decreasing cancer, strengthening bone, improving mood, and decreasing other disease processes. It is not necessary to go out and run a marathon immediately—or at all. Brisk walking for thirty minutes most days of the week can be very beneficial. Other aerobic exercises that offer similar benefits include jogging, swimming, bicycling, and water aerobics.

The key for exercise selection is to choose something that is enjoyable since that increases the probability it will become a routine. The current guidelines recommend 150 minutes of exercise per week. Five days at thirty minutes per day would help to attain that goal. In addition to aerobic exercise, strength training with weights and resistance can increase flexibility, strength, and balance. I am a huge proponent of exercise and I think that most if not all can reap some benefits from it.

Not a fan of standard exercise? Raking leaves, mowing the grass, and gardening are also beneficial. For the menopausal woman who is just getting started with an exercise program, I recommend that you begin slowly and over time increase your routine.

At this stage in life, it is important for women to be cognizant of how they feel and to remember that the old adage of "no pain no gain'" is no longer recommended. During exercise, gentle stretching should be appreciated but pushing yourself to extremes will only lead to injury.

The benefits of exercise outweigh the risks. Weight gain is common during the aging process. Women typically gain one pound per year from age forty through sixty-five. Regular exercise helps to prevent this weight gain. Hormonal changes during menopause cause a redistribution of weight from the typical "pear" shape that women have during the younger years to the more "apple" shape that mimics the weight distribution found in men. Apple-shaped weight distribution (fat distribution concentrated around the waist) is associated with an increase in certain diseases. The apple shape increases the risk of heart disease, high blood pressure, diabetes, and certain cancers. Risks of cancers such as breast, colon, and uterine are reduced with regular exercise. It is additionally established that the risk of osteoporosis, diabetes, heart disease, and hypertension are also decreased.

Some menopausal symptoms are reduced with regular exercise. Women who exercise regularly tend to have fewer hot flashes and tend to have less insomnia. They also tend to be calmer. The overall feeling of well-being is an undeniable benefit of regular exercise.

It is never too late to begin to take care of ourselves. There is no time like the present. Caring for ourselves through every stage of life—even the stages that feel uncomfortable and foreign at first—should be a priority. For the aging woman, exercise and a healthy diet are ways she can embrace the menopausal changes and lead her life in a more confident and vibrant direction.

"My task is not to seek for love, but to seek and find all the barriers within myself that I have built against it."

—RUMI

CHAPTER 11

THE DOCTOR'S VISIT

Many of my patients come to visit me with menopausal complaints and want some kind of relief. My goal is to treat the entire patient and not just her menopausal symptoms. I believe that the perimenopausal/menopausal transition is not just a one-stop shop and should include a more holistic approach. Oftentimes during the reproductive years, the obstetrician/gynecologist is the only provider that a patient has. I believe that around the menopausal transition if a woman does not have a primary care provider it is time to get one. Health challenges associated with aging require that a woman obtain the expertise of her primary care provider in addition to her obstetrician and gynecologist. Although the entire female body is affected by menopause some of the most common diseases that affect menopausal women are heart disease, breast cancer, colorectal cancer, and osteoporosis.

SCREENING GUIDELINES FOR THE PATIENT FORTY YEARS OLD AND OLDER

CERVICAL CANCER SCREENING

Cervical cancer screening is performed via the Pap smear. This testing should begin at age twenty-one. The traditional Pap smear has been around since the 1940s and has changed since its inception. The current technology not only screens for cervical cancer cells but also screens for the HPV, human papillomavirus, which is the precursor for the abnormal cells. The frequency of the Pap test originally recommended to be performed annually has been extended in many cases. Talk with your medical provider regarding the frequency of your testing. Guidelines now suggest that Pap testing can be discontinued between sixty-five and seventy years of age depending on a woman's history.

The pelvic exam done to examine the internal organs is done along with the Pap smear. I have found that most of my patients appreciate having their Pap and pelvic exams done annually because there are other topics they want to discuss. As with any concern a woman should have a conversation with her provider as to how often she needs to be tested.

BREAST CANCER SCREENING

Although the experts disagree on the monthly breast self-exam, I still encourage routine self-breast exams. I have seen instances in which women or their partners have discovered the breast abnormality. Part of the routine gynecological examination includes the breast examination. For women at regular risk for breast cancer, the guidelines recommend mammograms beginning at age forty, which is a change from the previous recommendation of age thirty-five. Thereafter in regular-risk patients, mammograms are generally recommended every one to two years. There is still some expert disagreement on the frequency of mammograms in the forty- to-forty-nine-year-old age group, so women should discuss this with their medical provider.

It is established that genetics plays a role in the development of breast cancer, so genetic testing may be appropriate for some patients. One of the things we as providers fail to do is to discuss breast cancer prevention. We frequently discuss breast cancer discovery using mammography, but we fail to discuss breast cancer prevention. Regular exercise several times per week can decrease the risk of breast cancer by 10 to 20 percent. Additionally, breast cancer risk also can be decreased by the consumption of cruciferous vegetables including broccoli, cauliflower and kale.

COLORECTAL CANCER SCREENING

Of late, colon cancer has been occurring in patients younger than age forty. The newest guidelines recommend screening begin at age forty-five instead of the previous age of fifty and every five years thereafter in regular-risk patients. Patients at risk for colon cancer include those with a strong family history of colon cancer or colonic polyps. With the removal of colonic polyps, colon cancer can be prevented. Additional risk factors for colon cancer include a low fiber diet, age over fifty and a sedentary lifestyle.

The gold standard test for colon cancer is the colonoscopy where a scope is inserted into the colon as a visual test for the disease. Light sedation is used.

OSTEOPOROSIS SCREENING
Osteoporosis, the thinning of bones, is more common in certain groups of women. Caucasian and Asian women have an increased risk of osteoporosis as do thin women, cigarette smokers and those with a history of fractures. In an average-risk patient, the usual age for a DEXA (dual energy X-ray absorptiometry) scan to evaluate the bone thickness is sixty-five.

BLOOD PRESSURE SCREENING
Blood pressures should be checked at routine physical exams. There are new guidelines for blood pressure measurement and even lower blood pressures than originally thought are considered more optimal. Blood pressures from 130-139/80-89 should be evaluated by your provider. If other disease processes are present such as diabetes, heart disease, or kidney disease then blood pressures should be managed more closely.

CHOLESTEROL SCREENING

Cholesterol screening includes testing total cholesterol, LDL (low density lipoprotein), HDL (high density lipoprotein) and triglycerides. LDL is considered the 'negative' cholesterol so the lower the number the better, while HDL is termed the 'good' cholesterol and the higher the number the better. The recommended age for cholesterol testing is age fifty. This blood test recommended every five years for the average risk patient should be taken after overnight fasting. For patients with other disease processes such as hypertension, diabetes, obesity and a strong family history of heart disease there should be consideration for more frequent testing.

DIABETES SCREENING

For average-risk patients, screening for diabetes mellitus should begin at age forty-five with testing every three years. Other risk factors such as hypertension, kidney disease and family history necessitate more frequent testing.

LUNG CANCER SCREENING

Screening for lung cancer is typically done with a chest x-ray and/or a computed tomography (CT). Patients in the high-risk group include those with a thirty-pack per year smoking history and those over age fifty-five.

SKIN CANCER EXAM

Women who are high risk for skin cancer include those who have a history of skin cancer and those who spend frequent time in the sun. Other risk factors include a family history of skin cancer and those with a weakened immune system. For women who find themselves in the high-risk category, it may be prudent to obtain regular whole skin evaluations.

THYROID TESTING
The thyroid gland should be examined during the physical exam. A thyroid blood test can be done especially if the examination of the thyroid gland is abnormal.

IMMUNIZATIONS
Current guidelines recommend an influenza shot annually. A pneumococcal vaccine may also be recommended for patients over the age of sixty-five or with certain respiratory issues. Shingles vaccine may be recommended beginning at age fifty along with a tetanus/diphtheria/pertussis (Tdap). Tdap boosters are recommended every ten years.

While all of these screenings and tests may seem overwhelming, I want to stress that menopause is a normal and natural progression of life. Often, these tests are a part of preventative care and not necessarily done because all women of a certain age have all of these issues. As a doctor, I treat the entire patient. We evaluate nutritional habits and exercise programs. We look at the woman's mental well-being and other lifestyle factors. When necessary I prescribe medication to assist the menopausal woman. I find that the holistic approach is the best way to treat a patient and I encourage the involvement of her other healthcare providers.

The involvement of her other medical providers allows for a more continuous and holistic approach. As providers, we want to be cognizant of not just the physical effects of menopause but the spiritual, emotional and mental as well. Only with the full picture can we treat the full patient—and the full picture is even more important when medications are necessary. We will discuss medications specific to menopausal women in the next chapter.

"Imperfect action is better than perfect inaction."

—HARRY S. TRUMAN

CHAPTER 12

MENOPAUSE AND MEDICATION

"I am looking for a medication that is not too extreme. I heard that hormones are not good for you."

There are not many more controversial areas in medicine than menopausal hormone therapy (MHT). At one time it was thought that hormone therapy should be routinely used for all women and in all cases. We have learned this is not the case and we have adjusted our thinking. Menopausal hormone therapies are medications that replace the decreasing hormones and are used to treat menopausal symptoms.

Hormone therapy comes in different formulations including systemic therapy and local therapy. Systemic hormone therapy comes in the form of pills, patches, creams, gels, and sprays that deliver hormone therapy to the entire system by being absorbed by the entire body. Localized hormone therapy is delivered directly to the vagina and treats the localized vaginal dryness. Local therapies come in the form of creams, tablets, vaginal pills, or rings and have little to no systemic absorption.

Before we delve into the benefits and risks of MHT, there is a landmark study that merits discussion. This study sponsored by the National Institutes of Health termed the Women's Health Initiative (WHI) enrolled over 160,000 postmenopausal women across the United States between the ages of fifty and seventy-nine. Some of the most common diseases affecting postmenopausal women include cardiovascular disease, breast and colorectal cancer, and osteoporosis. Initiated in 1991, the study goals were to employ strategies to decrease the incidence of these diseases in postmenopausal women (1).

The three arms of the study included the clinical arm, the observational study, and the community prevention study. There were significant findings from the WHI. One of the most significant was that estrogen-plus-progestin therapy in the postmenopausal patient increased the risk for heart disease, stroke, blood clots, breast cancer, and dementia. However, in the estrogen-only study, it was found that there was only a marginal increase in the risk of stroke and blood clots while there was no increase in the risk of heart attacks and breast cancer (2).

The other findings of the WHI showed that a low-fat diet did not significantly reduce the risk of breast cancer, heart disease, stroke, and colorectal cancer, but it may reduce the risk of ovarian cancer (3). Additionally, the calcium and vitamin D trial showed that these supplements provided a modest benefit in preserving bone mass and decreasing hip fractures in older women. As a result of the WHI findings, some changes in women's health were made.

No longer do we employ hormone replacement therapy (HRT) for the treatment of heart disease as we did prior to the WHI. With the concern of increased risk of breast cancer, we now require that women have a normal mammogram prior to initiating HRT and we employ its use for the shortest amount of time using the lowest required dose to diminish the symptoms of menopause.

MENOPAUSAL HORMONE THERAPY REGIMENS
The goal of menopausal hormone therapy (MHT) is to decrease the menopausal related symptoms in an attempt to improve the quality of life for the perimenopausal and menopausal woman. Included in the MHT is the use of unopposed estrogen or estrogen alone and combination therapy with estrogen and progestin. Of note, unopposed estrogen therapy as its name implies does not include progestin therapy. Unopposed estrogen therapy should not be used in a woman with a uterus since unopposed estrogen (estrogen without progestin) increases the risk of endometrial cancer. Endometrial cancer, cancer of the lining of the uterus, is a common gynecological cancer. Also of note, MHT replacement in general uses progestin, which is the synthetic formulation of progesterone, the natural form. Other formulations include estrogens and SERMs. A SERM (selective estrogen receptor modulator) can be utilized along with estrogen or as a stand-alone medication. A SERM is a designer drug that provides the benefits of estrogen to certain

parts of the body while at the same time reducing the side effects of estrogen to other parts of the body.

GENERALIZED GUIDELINES FOR MHT USAGE
The decision to use MHT should be an individual one between a woman and her healthcare provider. There is no place for a one-size-fits-all approach because every woman is different. A caveat employed by most providers is to use the smallest dose possible to alleviate the symptoms while at the same time minimizing the side effects. Of note, not all women react the same to the same medication formulation. One MHT regimen may work well for one woman but not for another. Prior to beginning a patient on MHT, I take a complete history including personal and family history and I use lab work in making my decision. The standard recommendation for the duration of MHT usage has been five years or less and not to use past age sixty. However, I have found that some patients past age sixty are still having some menopausal symptoms and want to continue to use MHT. Experts from societies such as the American College of Obstetricians and Gynecologists agree that the use of MHT should be individualized and not discontinued because of age but rather can be used if the benefits outweigh the risks (4).

ESTROGEN THERAPY
Estrogen therapy is available in many forms. These formulations include oral (pills), a transdermal patch (worn on

the skin), a vaginal ring, vaginal creams, a vaginal tablet, sprays, and creams. Typically the route of administration of any MHT is based upon patient preference, cost of the medication, and medication availability. I prefer not to use the oral estrogen formulations in my practice secondary to the increases in liver and gallbladder disease caused by the oral formulation. Additionally, the oral formulation can decrease the amount of available testosterone in the bloodstream, which is another reason I prefer not to use it. The vaginal estrogen formulations help to alleviate vaginal dryness with little to no systemic absorption, hence progestin may not be required in this instance in protection of the uterine lining.

PROGESTIN THERAPY

As mentioned, if a woman still has her uterus and is considering MHT, progestin therapy should be added in order to decrease the incidence of endometrial cancer. Progestin is the synthetic form of progesterone, the natural hormone. I prefer to use the natural progesterone when I can as opposed to the synthetic formulation since natural progesterone does not cause the elevated cholesterol and triglyceride levels. Progestin formulations also come in oral, topical, and vaginal forms. Since other parts of the body have progesterone receptors, using the natural form can help with other menopausal symptoms such as insomnia and depression.

SERMs (Selective Estrogen Receptor Modulators)

This novel class of drugs is used to provide the benefits of estrogen to specific parts of the body while decreasing the risks of it to other parts of the body. SERMs are used to reduce osteoporosis and to decrease the risk of breast cancer in a select group of women. One of the SERMs is used to treat moderate vaginal dryness and atrophy of the external genitalia. Another SERM combined with estrogen is available for the treatment of menopausal hot flashes and to prevent osteoporosis. A progestin is not necessary with this medication and is appropriate for the patient who cannot tolerate the side effects of progestin therapy. A significant side effect of the SERM is the increased risk of blood clots in the leg known as deep venous thrombosis, or DVTs.

Potential Side Effects of MHT

Typical side effects of estrogen usage include breast tenderness and vaginal bleeding. In the patient who still has a uterus, the combination of estrogen-progestin therapy can cause a resumption of vaginal bleeding. Mood swings, depression, and bloating are sometimes seen with progestin therapy. SERMs can increase the risk of blood clots in the blood vessels. There are some women who MHT is not recommended for. These women are those with a personal history of breast cancer, coronary heart disease, and a history of a blood clot in the blood vessels such as that occurs in a stroke, leg clot, or pulmonary embolism (blood clot in the lung). Other contraindications or reasons not to use MHT include active liver disease, any unexplained vaginal bleeding, and any woman with a history of a mini-stroke (transient ischemic attack).

NONHORMONAL TREATMENTS

There are options for women who choose not to use hormone therapy. Although they may not work as well as estrogen in the treatment of hot flashes, they do help in some instances and tend to work better than placebo. These include the class of antidepressants known as SSRIs, selective serotonin reuptake inhibitors. These drugs, while used to treat depression, can also minimize the hot flashes associated with menopause. One medication used as an anti-seizure drug can also relieve hot flashes. I am excited about a new product on the market with promising results that employs natural remedies to help combat menopausal symptoms.

COMPOUNDED MENOPAUSAL HORMONE THERAPY (CMHT)

The number of prescriptions being written for MHT decreased in the early 2000s when the initial findings of the WHI study were published. With the findings of the WHI study and the concerns regarding the side effects of standard treatment, physicians and scientists began to search for alternatives. Enter bioidentical hormone therapy (BioHRT). Bioidentical hormone replacement therapy refers to hormones with the same molecular structure as the hormones produced by the body. These products are custom compounded by compounding pharmacies, and their formulations are prescribed based upon hormonal blood levels, which are drawn prior to initiating therapy. The hormones that are typically compounded are estradiol, estrone and estriol, which are the three subtypes of estrogen. Additional compounded hormones include progesterone, testosterone, and dehydroepiandrosterone (DHEA). These compounds are derived from soy and plant extracts. While these products are not FDA approved nor regulated, there are state guidelines that regulate their production.

As women began to search for other options, the use of bioidentical hormones increased. I use bioidentical hormones, standard MHT, and the newer natural nonhormonal remedies in my practice. I like the idea that compounded medication comes from plant sources, which I feel are safer than animal sources, and I like to add other hormones such as testosterone into my patient's medication regimen. I appreciate being able to monitor patient progress using hormonal blood levels. Along with my compounded pharmacy, I am able to monitor a woman's progress with her bioidentical hormones.

Choosing the appropriate medication for a woman is an individualized one. A complete history and physical are obtained and blood work as needed.

An updated mammogram is obtained. My intent and goal is to treat the patient with the most appropriate medication for her to make the most of her menopausal transition.

The most common reason for using MHT is to treat the annoying menopausal symptoms. Medication is not for everyone, but having a great menopausal transition is!

"Resentment is like drinking poison and hoping it will kill your enemies."

—NELSON MANDELA

CHAPTER 13

THE BEST OF MENOPAUSE

PATIENT TESTIMONIALS FROM THE FABULOUS FOUR

I wanted patient input in preparing this manuscript. Who better to give an opinion regarding menopause than the ladies who have gone through it? What do they think? How has menopause positively affected their lives? What advice do they have for other women?

I call these women the fabulous four. Each one of them is at a different stage in their life. They come from different walks of life. They don't know one another, but they share the common experience of having gone through the menopausal transition. Their names have been edited to maintain anonymity, but they know who they are. I thank each and every one of them for their contribution to this manuscript. I wish them favor. I wish them good health. I wish them all the best of their menopausal transition!

PATIENT #1 – ANGELA K.

I like the fact that I am wiser and smarter than before menopause. I don't know if it is the change in my hormones or what, but I feel so much better about myself. As I go through my day, I realize that I have more of what it takes to handle life and all that it throws my way. I really like the person that I am becoming.

I would say to any perimenopausal woman about to go through it to remain active. I advise her to eat well and get lots of exercise. Sometimes I get so busy with the family and work that I forget to do those extra things to take care of myself. Take time to smell the roses and slow down. Value yourself. Have a day that is a self-care day and spend time pampering yourself. You deserve it. I am going right now to heed my advice and spoil myself!

PATIENT #2 – MAY P.
I never liked having menstrual periods. They seemed to always get in the way of my life. I was so glad when they stopped. I feel freer and now I am able to do those things that I couldn't when I was having periods. I am saving so much money because now I don't have to buy pads.

I would say to any woman about to go through it to make sure you take care of yourself. Be good to yourself. Even though some days you may wake up and not feel like doing something, do it anyway. Menopausal women need to take that extra care of themselves because of the changes that are going on in the body. Give yourself the extra nap, the extra workout. Get the extra hug from your family and friends. Simply, just love on yourself.

PATIENT #3 – SHELLY R.
For me, the best part of menopause is having a doctor who is willing to go through it with you. I am able to go to my doctor and she listens to me. She understood what I was saying and I didn't feel like I was crazy. My doctor told me that my feelings were valid. She helped me to come up with a hormone program that would help me to feel better. She also helped me to realize that I am not in this thing alone because there are other women out there who are experiencing this transition. I have been praying a lot so all this has made me closer to God.

The advice that I have for women is to seek help. The feelings that you are having are real and not in your head. Do not sit by quietly and suffer in silence. Get a good doctor or therapist to help you sort out your feelings and thoughts. Remember that you are not alone. It is okay to seek help. I did and I am better for it!

PATIENT #4 – LYNN C.
My sexual appetite is better since I have gone through menopause. I want sex so much more now than before. I don't have to worry about getting pregnant now. My children are grown and out of the house, and most times, it's just me and my husband. We can walk around naked if we want and not worry about a thing. I have hit a milestone age and I like it.

To my younger counterparts I would say have fun! Take all of this in stride because the time will come when you will go through it. Remember that it is a phase in life. You can remember what you used to do all day long, but so what? Some things you cannot do any more, but that is okay because you have a new lease on life. Make sure that you have a good support system and people around you that help you. Explore your new life. See what adventures it holds. Don't let menopause stop you—keep on moving!

"All journeys outward ultimately lead to the journey inward where everything I seek already exists and awaits my joyous acceptance."

—AUTHOR UNKNOWN

THE MENOPAUSAL QUIZ

HOW MUCH DO YOU KNOW ABOUT MENOPAUSE?
Before becoming a physician, I was a middle school science and high school biology teacher in South Bend, Indiana. I learned to love knowledge and the quest for knowledge. Much to the dismay of my students, I enjoyed testing their knowledge with regular pop quizzes. Although they did not appreciate the pop quizzes, I hope they were made better because of it. The teacher in me could not help but to write a self-test to see how much you learned after reading this book. No one is keeping score but you.

1. The average age of menopause in the United States is _____.
    a. 65
    b. 52.4
    c. 40
    d. 58.6

2. Menopause is defined as the complete cessation of menses for _____.
    a. One year
    b. Two years
    c. Six months
    d. Eighteen months

3. Hormones are derived from _____.
   a. Testosterone
   b. Estrogen
   c. Cholesterol
   d. Progesterone

4. At the time of puberty, what is the usual order of development?
   a. Breast development, pubic hair development, axillary hair development, menses
   b. Pubic hair development, axillary hair development, menses, breast development
   c. Menses, breast development, axillary hair development, pubic hair development
   d. Breast development, axillary hair development, pubic hair development, menses

5. Vaginal folds called _____ help to increase friction during sexual intercourse.
   a. Spider veins
   b. Genitalia
   c. Rugae
   d. Mons pubis

6. What hormone is important in the sleep-wake cycle?

    a. Pancreas
    b. Interleukin 12
    c. Glucose
    d. Melatonin

7. What percentage of women experience the menopausal hot flash?

    a. 5 percent
    b. 12 percent
    c. 40 percent
    d. 80 percent

8. Which organ functions as the orchestrator of our movements?

    a. Liver
    b. Brain
    c. Ears
    d. Pharyngeal tube

9. Which one of these factors if present DECREASES the risk of heart disease in women?

    a. Sedentary lifestyle
    b. Exercise
    c. Cigarette smoking
    d. Hypertension (high blood pressure)

10. The largest organ of the body is the _____.
    a. Heart
    b. Pancreas
    c. Pituitary gland
    d. Skin

11. Which of the following occurs in the digestive system during menopause?
    a. Incomplete digestion of food
    b. An increase in the good bacteria
    c. A shift of body fat to the neck region
    d. A decrease in farting

12. Severe thinning of the bone is termed _____ and can lead to debilitating fractures.
    a. Osteoporosis
    b. Perineal bulge
    c. Uveitis
    d. Endometritis

13. Which of the following is NOT a component of the immune system?
    a. Bone marrow
    b. Spleen
    c. White blood cells
    d. Cornea

14. _____ are compounds that are derived from plants and mimic estrogen's actions.

    a. Androgens
    b. Phytoestrogens
    c. Capsaicin
    d. Latex cloths

15. What percentage of women are plagued with urinary incontinence?

    a. 10 percent
    b. 20 percent
    c. 40 percent
    d. 80 percent

16. Which of the following worsens the brain changes that can be seen during menopause?

    a. Cigarette smoking
    b. Yoga
    c. Exercise
    d. Good nutrition

17. Which of the following does NOT increase the risk of osteoporosis?

    a. Thyroid disease
    b. Cigarette smoking
    c. Thin body habitus
    d. Exercise

18. What percentage of the menopausal diet should be comprised of fats?

    a. 8 percent
    b. 10 percent
    c. 30 percent
    d. 70 percent

19. Changes in fat distribution in the mid-section of menopausal women have been likened to what fruit?

    a. Apple
    b. Banana
    c. Orange
    d. Strawberry

20. The new guidelines recommend that colorectal cancer screening begin at age____.

    a. 40
    b. 45
    c. 50
    d. 55

TEST ANSWER KEY

1. b	8. b	15. c
2. a	9. b	16. a
3. c	10. d	17. d
4. a	11. a	18. c
5. c	12. a	19. a
6. d	13. d	20. b
7. d	14. b	

MY MENOPAUSAL GUIDE

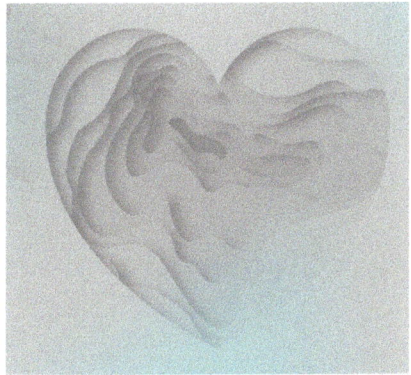

I have created this menopausal guide so that you can ask and answer the tough questions for yourself. Below I've included a chart to rank symptoms you may be having, along with questions to help you better understand the changes your body is undergoing. You can fill it out here or on a separate sheet of paper, but answering these questions is a great start to not only better understanding your body but preparing for conversations with your doctor on how to manage and treat symptoms.

MY SYMPTOMS

Please rank each symptom below based upon the level of severity.

	Absent	Mild	Moderate	Severe
Fibrocystic breast				
Weight gain				
Irregular periods				
Hot flashes				
Dry skin/hair				
Anxiety				
Depression				
Night sweats				
Vaginal dryness				
Headaches				
Irritability				
Mood swings				
Breast tenderness				
Insomnia				
Cramps				
Fluid retention				
Fatigue				
Loss of memory				
Incontinence				
Arthritis				
Harder to climax				
Decreased libido				
Hair loss				

MENOPAUSAL WORKBOOK

At what age did I begin to notice menopausal symptoms?

_____
_____
_____

What were some of the symptoms I first noticed that alerted me that things were changing?

_____
_____
_____

If I were to sum up this transitional change, is it more bad or good?

_____
_____
_____

Name three positive things about the change that I have experienced.

_____
_____
_____

Name three negative things about the change that I have experienced.

_____

_____

_____

What have I found that seems to worsen the symptoms?

_____

_____

_____

What have I found that seems to make the symptoms better?

_____

_____

_____

How can I improve my diet?

_____

_____

_____

Am I getting enough exercise?

_____

_____

_____

What are my life stressors?

_____

_____

_____

Do I need to see a doctor?

_____

_____

_____

Now that I have read this book, what changes am I going to implement?

_____

_____

_____

_____

_____

_____

_____

_____

_____

_____

_____

AFTERWORD

CELEBRATE THE UNIQUENESS OF YOU

As I wrote this book, I was constantly reminded of one of the reasons that I elected to become a physician. I have always had a fascination with the human body. It is a marvel and a wonder. Most days when we awaken, our minds are so preoccupied with plans for the day that we rarely consider the intricacies and nuances that were responsible for our waking that day. There are a vast number of factors that went into our being able to open our eyes to begin the day. Your day. Your limited number of days on earth. We are uniquely created just like snowflakes. It is beyond imagination that never has there been, is there, or will there ever be another person like me or like you—EVER. We are complex creatures and that is what makes us so fascinating. We are given one chance to live this life and I wish you very few regrets. I want you to grab all of life that is yours to grab without letting the menopausal change stop you.

I wrote this book so that women entering menopause have a reliable resource to navigate through the change. I hope it has helped you. I want you to experience the joys of the menopausal change. I want you to embrace who you are and to celebrate the uniqueness of you. Be in touch with yourself. Acknowledge that you are an imperfect being. Be vulnerable because out of your vulnerability comes your strength and courage. Realize that you don't have to be strong every minute of every day. Be true to yourself and realize that menopause is just a phase of life. The body changes are inevitable, but I hope this book helps to lighten the load of those changes. I hope that you meet this new you with everything that you need to soar. Bask in the fact that there will never be another you. Be unpredictable. Be bold. Be dynamic. Be confident. Be beautiful. You are GOD's unique gift to the world. There will NEVER be another you. Celebrate your uniqueness.

ACKNOWLEDGMENTS

I want to thank Dr. Draion Burch for seeing this book in me. Once you acknowledged that I was a writer, I took it from there. You recognized my writing skills even though I had suppressed them at age sixteen to pursue a career in medicine. You knew that the desire and talent were still there. Thank you for pushing me to excellence.

I want to thank my husband, James H. Kerns, III, for loving me and supporting me along this journey and giving me what I needed to get it done.

To GOD, I could not have done it without your guidance and wisdom. I hope that I am living my life in such a way that you are glorified.

REFERENCES

1. "Design of the Women's Health Initiative Clinical Trial and Observational Study. The Women's Health Initiative Study Group. Control Clinical Trials." 1998: 19(1): 61-109.

2. Manson, J. E., J. Hsia, K. C. Johnson, J. E. Rossouw, A. R. Assaf, N. L. Lasser, et al. "Estrogen Plus Progestin and the Risk of Coronary Heart Disease." *New England Journal of Medicine*. 2003; 349(6): 523-524.

3. Grady D., S. M. Rubin, D. B. Petiti, S. Fox, D. Black, B. Ettinger, et al. "Hormone Therapy To Prevent Disease and Prolong Life in Postmenopausal Women." *Annals of Internal Medicine*. 1992; 117(12): 1016-37.

4. American College of Obstetricians and Gynecologists. Practice Bulletin 141. 2014: 1-8.

ABOUT THE AUTHOR

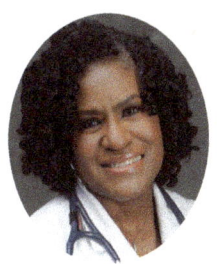

Dr. Barbara Ann Hannah, board-certified obstetrician and gynecologist, knows the woes of the menopausal and perimenopausal woman. She is passionate about helping these women transition into menopause with confidence and vibrancy. Dr. Bobbi, as she is affectionately known to her patients, wants to arm women with the knowledge they need to make sound and healthful choices as they transition through the change. She hopes this book fosters a positive perspective for women and their loved ones regarding this new phase of life and that menopause is no longer seen as a dreadful time.

Dr. Bobbi is in private practice and is the owner and CEO of Women's Center/HealthCare Physicians as well as a partner at Advanced HealthCare Associates in the Detroit metro area. She is married to James H. Kerns, III, whom she met at her beloved alma mater, Kentucky State University.

Learn more at dr.bobbiOBGYN.com

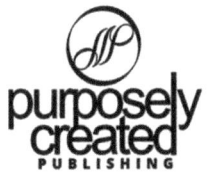

CREATING DISTINCTIVE BOOKS
WITH INTENTIONAL RESULTS

We're a collaborative group of creative masterminds with a mission to produce high-quality books to position you for monumental success in the marketplace.

Our professional team of writers, editors, designers, and marketing strategists work closely together to ensure that every detail of your book is a clear representation of the message in your writing.

Want to know more?
Write to us at info@publishyourgift.com
or call (888) 949-6228

Discover great books, exclusive offers, and more at
www.PublishYourGift.com

Connect with us on social media

@publishyourgift

www.ingramcontent.com/pod-product-compliance
Ingram Content Group UK Ltd.
Pitfield, Milton Keynes, MK11 3LW, UK
UKHW020243240426
12048UKWH00026B/1580